Primary Immune Deficiencies
Made Simple

Handbook for Practicing Pediatricians, Physicians, and Medical Students

Primary Immune Deficiencies
Made Simple

Handbook for Practicing Pediatricians, Physicians, and Medical Students

Sagar Bhattad

MBBS, MD (Pediatrics), DM (Pediatric Clinical Immunology and Rheumatology) (PGI Chd)

Consultant, Pediatric Immunologist and Rheumatologist
Aster CMI Hospital, New Airport Road
Sahakara Nagar, Hebbal, Bengaluru-560092, Karnataka

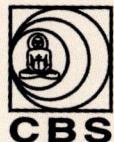

CBS

CBS Publishers & Distributors Pvt Ltd

New Delhi • Bengaluru • Chennai • Kochi • Kolkata • Mumbai
Hyderabad • Jharkhand • Nagpur • Patna • Pune • Uttarakhand

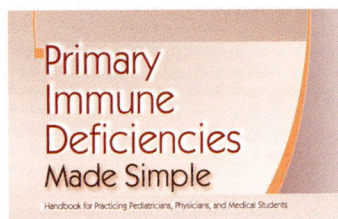

Primary Immune Deficiencies Made Simple
Handbook for Practicing Pediatricians, Physicians, and Medical Students

ISBN: 978-93-90158-96-6

First Edition: 2021
Reprint 2021

Published by Satish Kumar Jain and produced by Varun Jain for

CBS Publishers & Distributors Pvt Ltd
4819/XI Prahlad Street, 24 Ansari Road, Daryaganj, New Delhi 110 002, India
Ph: 011-23289259, 23266861, 23266867   Fax: 011-23243014
Website: www.cbspd.com   e-mail: delhi@cbspd.com; cbspubs@airtelmail.in

Corporate Office: 204 FIE, Industrial Area, Patparganj, Delhi 110 092, India
Ph: 011-49344934   Fax: 011-49344935   e-mail: publishing@cbspd.com; publicity@cbspd.com

Branches

- **Bengaluru:** Seema House 2975, 17th Cross, K.R. Road, Banasankari 2nd Stage, Bengaluru 560 070, Karnataka, India
  Ph: +91-80-26771678/79   Fax: +91-80-26771680   e-mail: bangalore@cbspd.com
- **Chennai:** 7, Subbaraya Street, Shenoy Nagar, Chennai 600 030, Tamil Nadu, India
  Ph: +91-44-26680620, 26681266   Fax: +91-44-42032115   e-mail: chennai@cbspd.com
- **Kochi:** 42/1325, 1326, Power House Road, Opposite KSEB, Power House, Ernakulum-682018, Kochi, Kerala, India
  Ph: +91-484-4059061-67   Fax: +91-484-4059065   e-mail: kochi@cbspd.com
- **Kolkata:** 6/B, Ground Floor, Rameswar Shaw Road, Kolkata-700 014 (West Bengal), India
  Ph: +91-33-22891126, 22891127, 22891128   e-mail: kolkata@cbspd.com
- **Mumbai:** PWD Shed, Gala No. 25/26, Ramchandra Bhatt Marg, Next JJ Hospital Gate No. 2
  Opp. Union Bank of India, Noorbaug, Mumbai-400009, Maharashtra, India
  Ph: +91-22-66661880/89   e-mail: mumbai@cbspd.com

Representatives

• **Hyderabad**	0-9885175004	• **Jharkhand**	0-9811541605	• **Nagpur**	0-9421945513
• **Patna**	0-9334159340	• **Pune**	0-9623451994	• **Uttarakhand**	0-9716462459

Printed at: Nutech Print Services, Faridabad, Haryana, India

Foreword

I consider it a unique honour, and a singular privilege, to be asked to write this note of introduction for our erstwhile student and now a dear colleague Dr Sagar Badrinarayan Bhattad.

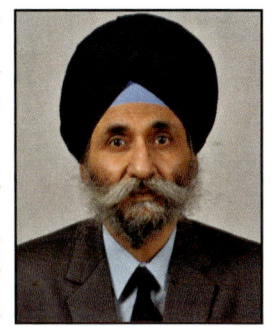

Sagar completed his residency in pediatrics in our department in December 2013. He topped his batch and was awarded the coveted Silver Medal for excellence in the subject. His MD thesis paper on childhood lupus (under guidance of Prof Amit Rawat) was selected for Maj. Gen. Amir Chand Gold Medal as the best published paper amongst all MD/MS students in the institute for that year. This prize is one of the most prestigious awards in our institute.

Sagar had the courage (and the foresight) to apply for the first batch of DM in Pediatric Clinical Immunology and Rheumatology that had been initiated at our institute in January 2014. And this at a time when there were several other well-established DM programmes running in our department. He completed the course with flying colors in December 2016 and, in the process, set-up standards of training and patient care that we still follow. Having completed his training, he chose to move on nearer home and set-up a first-rate service in Pediatric Immunology and Rheumatology at Bengaluru. This service is now widely perceived to be one of the finest such efforts in South India.

'Primary Immune Deficiencies Made Simple' is a compendium of short essays on common primary immunodeficiency disorders that we encounter (and often miss) in our clinical practice. I have no hesitation in stating that this would soon become a 'ready reckoner' for all pediatricians and physicians in our country. The book reflects Sagar's own insight, experience and perspective on diagnosis and management of such patients who, unfortunately, often have to struggle for long periods before even getting to know what is wrong with them. Simplicity of concept and clarity of thought are the hallmarks of this book.

'Primary Immune Deficiencies Made Simple' is a very welcome initiative by one of our brightest students. I wish him all success!

Prof Surjit Singh
MD; DCH (Lon.); FRCP (Lon.); FRCPCH (Lon.); FAMS

Head, Department of Pediatrics and
Chief, Allergy Immunology Unit
Advanced Pediatrics Centre
Post Graduate Institute of Medical Education and Research
Chandigarh, India-160012

President
Asia Pacific Society for Immunodeficiencies (2020–2024)

Principal Investigator
Indian Council of Medical Research Centre
for Advanced Research in Primary Immunodeficiency Diseases
(2015–2020)

Vice-President
Indian Rheumatology Association (2017–2019)

Message...

Immunodeficiency disorders are a group of conditions that are not uncommon in pediatric practice. They often present with either severe, persistent, unusual or recurrent infections. Manifestations can be dramatic and early or subtle and delayed. While the awareness of these disorders is increasingly recognised in practice, advances in clinical training, laboratory sophistication and genetic analytic capabilities have helped clinicians define these conditions precisely. Once the diagnosis is clearly defined, therapeutic options have kept a rapid pace.

To partner with clinicians and to offer the best options of care, specialised immunologists are the need of the hour.

Dr Sagar Bhattad who has trained under the world renowned rheumato-logist/immunologist Dr Surjit Singh from the Post Graduate Institute, Chandigarh, has written a synopsis of immunodeficiency disorders seen in practice. This is peek into the immunologist's mind and the way he thinks through problems in practice. It will be of immense value to all pediatric clinicians.

With best wishes

Dr Jagdish Chinnappa
Cluster Head
Bangalore region, Manipal Hospitals
March 2020

Message...

This concise yet informative book on primary immune deficiency diseases authored by Dr Sagar Bhattad makes interesting reading to practicing pediatricians as well as postgraduates. It aptly fills in the long-felt gap in this area of clinical pediatrics. Suspecting PID is a job half completed. This book provides easy to follow, case-scenario based stepwise approach to the problem. Suspecting and initial screening for PID with available resources and timely referral as necessary will now happen and our children will benefit at large.

Dr Shashidhararao Nagabhushana
Visiting Professor, Rainbow Children Hospital, Bangalore
National Convener, Asthma Training Module of IAP

Message...

The foundation of Immunology were laid by Nobel Laureates Elie Metchnikoff (Father of Immunology—discovery of phagocytes and phagocytosis—1882), von Behring (serum therapy with neutralizing antibodies diphtheria and tetanus—1890) and Paul Ehrlich (blood smear staining for identifying different types of leucocytes, antiserum treatment for diphtheria and salvarsan for treatment of syphilis).

Immunology, as a pediatric subspeciality, has made great strides and progressed to unravel the mysteries of a plethora of inherited and acquired immunodeficiency states at all sites of immunoprotective and defensive mechanisms deciphered at cellular and humoral components of T and B lymphocytes and macrophages.

Quoting the British novelist and poet David Herbert Lawrence (1885–1930) "What the eye doesn't see and the mind doesn't know, doesn't exist". Pediatricians of my generation, though they thought of the possibility of an underlying PID in children presenting as generalised molluscum contagiosum in a young child, in others with recurrent pyoderma, eczema, mucosal infections with rare organisms, disseminated tuberculosis caused by BCG bacilli in live vaccine, they reached a dead end. Many such children with recurrent infections had finally succumbed to their fate termed genetics for want of diagnostic facilities and adequately trained subspecialists.

Primary Immunodeficiency Disorders (PIDs) in children, once considered rare, are no longer considered rare. Rightly, Dr Sagar Bhattad, Pediatric Immunologist, trained by Prof. (Dr) Surjit Singh of Advanced Pediatric Center, PGIMER, Chandigarh, India has begun his basic treatise–"*Handbook on Primary Immune Deficiencies–Made Simple*" with a positive approach and statement—"Eyes see only what mind knows", thus making the primary objective crystal clear. He has made a very important statement that pediatric residents in PGIMER, Chandigarh, would suspect and go on to diagnose these "no longer rare" entities on a day-to-day basis due to the important thrust given in training by one of the foremost and internationally known pediatric immunologists, Dr Surjit Singh.

All medical trainees and practitioners are told to keep 'open' mind, ears (history taking) and eyes (observation) whenever infants and children present with infections fulfilling the acronym 'SPUR' (S-Serious/Severe; P-Prolonged and/or Persistent in spite of appropriate treatment; U-Unusual agents; R-Recurrent) to suspect an underlying PID state. Though this is extremely relevant, it is also to be appreciated that PIDs can be suspected and diagnosed in the presence of a family history of deaths following infections in family members and siblings and in looking for a few specific "noninfectious signs" like unexplained persistent lymphadenopathy, eczema, etc., and thus need to be referred for specialist evaluation.

All current well-trained pediatric immunologists like Dr Sagar Bhattad have now a significant number of referred PID states from pediatric centers which could have been diagnosed earlier, if the importance of the above-mentioned noninfectious signs were given due consideration in the referring centers. Hence, Dr Sagar Bhattad, from his vast clinical experience from a large number of Childhood PIDs, has realized that it is high time to give adequate emphasis in training of pediatric trainees as well as practicing pediatricians by bringing out a tailor made, comprehensive, easily readable and uncomplicated handbook with the following objectives:

1. Elicit appropriate history of infections with 'SPUR' characteristics and deaths due to infections in the child, siblings and family members.
2. Understand and recognize the vital 'signs and symptoms' of infections pointing to the presence of a possible underlying 'PID' state.
3. Understand and recognize vital and specific "noninfectious signs and symptoms" distinctive of different inherited PID states.
4. Consult in house immunologist early to plan and investigate for PID without delay or refer to such a consultant nearby.
5. Counsel parents regarding the condition, need for special investigations to diagnose and the importance of early institution of appropriate treatment measures.
6. Recognize secondary causes of acquired secondary causes of deranged immunological function either due to infections or drugs or both.

I am privileged to know Dr Sagar Bhattad's expertise and work in this area and listen to his lucid and illustrative case presentations of PID conditions in infants and children since mid 2000. I am glad that he has taken up this commendable job to give new life to these unfortunate children with

PID states and hope to their parents. I am sure his primary objectives will bring in the desired orientation of the pediatric trainees and practitioners. I congratulate him for embarking on this ambitious project solely for early referral and work-up of these children to be cured of their PID and his mentor Dr Surjit singh for having trained such a competent and ideal pediatric immunologist.

Dr S Srinivasan
MD, DCH
Director, Professor and Head (Retd)
Department of Pediatrics, JIPMER, Pondicherry
Adjunct Professor
Department of Pediatrics
Mehta Multispeciality Hospital, Chennai

Message...

The book written by Dr Sagar Bhattad on primary immune deficiencies is a simple, informative, educative and easy to understand book. This book contains mainly basics of primary immune deficiencies and as many case scenarios which we come across our practice. These are often missed because of lack of orientation towards primary immunodeficiencies. This book would help to sensitize medical students, postgraduates and practicing pediatricians for early recognition and confirmation by basic tests and early referral, which will go a long way in improving the quality of life and longevity of these unfortunate children.

I congratulate Dr Sagar Bhattad for this innovative book.

Dr Bhaskar Shenoy
Head, Department of Paediatrics
Manipal Hospital
Bangalore

Preface

I was trained in the field of pediatric immunology and the science of primary immune deficiency diseases at the prestigious Post Graduate Institute of Medical Education and Research (PGIMER), Chandigarh. "Eyes see only what mind knows"—pediatric residents at PGIMER would diagnose immune deficiencies on a day-to-day basis; thanks to the department of immunology, excellent laboratory facilities and the phenomenal mentorship of Prof Surjit Singh.

As I began my career in Bangalore, I quickly realized the challenges faced by practicing pediatricians and residents in medical colleges. They were keen on diagnosing immune deficiencies and would love to help children suffering from these diseases, but had unique challenges: (a) Lack of trained immunologist who could guide them, (b) lack of laboratory facilities. But the most important issue was the lack of availability of a handbook on immune deficiency. A handbook which described these diseases in a simple language, provided clinical insights and clinically relevant algorithms for diagnosis, avoiding all the jargon of complex terminology and molecular immunology.

This handbook is a sincere effort in this regard. It aims to provide a clinical insight to practicing pediatricians, physicians and especially to medical students who often are thrilled to diagnose these conditions. Case-based learning is one of the best ways to understand a difficult subject and this book describes several real-life cases and would make you say, "I have seen such a case/many such cases". This, however, by no means is a complete textbook of immunology and a list of such textbooks would be provided in the handbook for the interested readers.

I hope you enjoy reading this book and in the process help children and adults suffering from primary immune deficiency diseases.

Sagar Bhattad

Acknowledgments

I would like to thank Almighty and my parents for showering their blessings on me; my wife Prerna and daughter Prisha for their love and constant support.

I would like to dedicate this book to my mentor Prof Surjit Singh (Head, Department of Pediatrics, PGIMER, Chandigarh) and my alma mater PGIMER, Chandigarh. It was only because of his guidance and the training at this prestigious institute, I am in a position to write this book today.

I would like to thank Dr Chetan Ginigeri, Dr Harish Kumar, Dr Sudheer, Dr Ravi Kumar, Dr Stalin Ramprakash, and Dr Raghuram, my colleagues at Aster CMI Hospital for inspiring me to take up this task. Dr Chetan has been the driving force behind my YouTube videos on immune deficiency.

I would also like to thank Dr Avinash Sharma (Assistant Professor, Pediatric Immunology and Rheumatology, Rajendra Prasad Government Medical College, Tanda, Himachal Pradesh), my friend and colleague; and Dr Amit Rawat (Professor, Department of Pediatrics, PGIMER, Chandigarh) for proofreading the book and providing valuable inputs for the final and improved version of this book.

My special thanks to the medical residents whose eagerness to learn the science of immune deficiency provided me the energy to pen this book.

Most important of all, I would like to thank my patients, who have taught me and continue to teach me, the fascinating science of immunology. I sincerely hope this small contribution of mine, would lead to timely diagnosis and therapy in patients with primary immune deficiency.

Sagar Bhattad

Abbreviations

PID	: Primary immune deficiency
IEI	: Inborn errors of immunity
HIV	: Human immune deficiency virus
AIDS	: Acquired immune deficiency syndrome
NADPH oxidase	: Nicotinamide adenine dinucleotide phosphate hydrogen oxidase
CGD	: Chronic granulomatous disease
LAD	: Leukocyte adhesion defect
SCID	: Severe combined immune deficiency
MSMD	: Mendelian susceptibility to mycobacterial disease
XLA	: X-linked agammaglobulinemia
CVID	: Common variable immune deficiency
WAS	: Wiskott-Aldrich syndrome
IBD	: Inflammatory bowel disease
IVIg	: Intravenous immunogloblin
CBC	: Complete blood count
Hb	: Hemoglobin
TC	: Total white cell count
DC	: Differential white cell count
PC	: Platelet count
ANC	: Absolute neutrophil count
ALC	: Absolute lymphocyte count
MPV	: Mean platelet volume
LFT	: Liver function test
RFT	: Renal function test
NBT	: Nitroblue tetrazolium test
DHR	: Dihydrorhodamine test
NGS	: Next-generation sequencing
JMF	: Jeffrey Modell Foundation
IUIS	: International Union of Immunological Societies

Contents

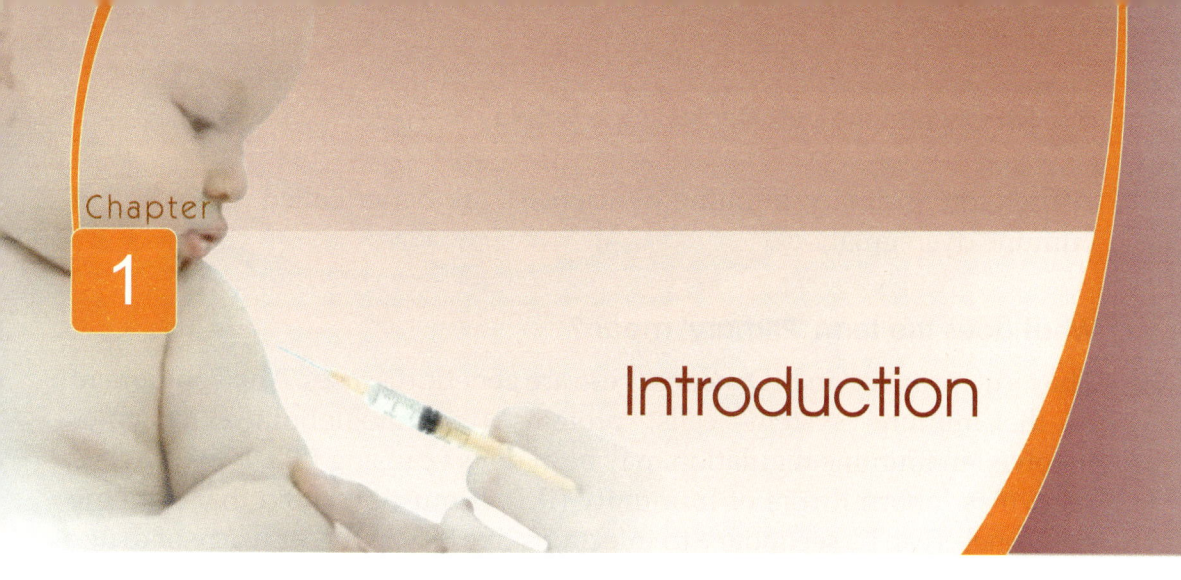

Introduction

> *Immune Deficiency Diseases are not rare!*
> *The Eyes See Only What the Mind Knows!*

Primary immune deficiencies (PID) are a group of heterogeneous disorders characterized by increased susceptibility to infections, autoimmunity, and malignancy due to a defect in the immune system.

The immune system is akin to an army that constantly protects us from our enemies. In this context, pathogenic microorganisms like bacteria, virus, and fungi can be presumed as our enemies and the white blood cells (neutrophils, lymphocytes) as the soldiers in the army of immune system that protect us. Absence or dysfunction of one of these cells would put an individual at unusually increased risk of infections, these conditions are called 'primary immune deficiencies.'

What are the functions of a healthy immune system?

1. Protection from invading microbes
2. Deletes autoreactive cells and prevents autoimmunity
3. Keeps a check on mutant cells and prevents cancers—*cancer surveillance*

A defect in immune system would therefore predispose an individual to

1. Increased risk of infections
2. Increased autoimmune diseases
3. Increased predisposition for malignancies

Therefore, primary immune deficiencies are better called 'disorders of immune dysregulation'.

What does the term 'Primary' mean?

The term 'primary' in PID means these are genetic diseases. Any component of the immune system—cells, proteins (immunoglobulins), enzymes involved in immune regulation may be at defect causing PID. PIDs are now known as Inborn Errors of Immunity (IEI). It must be noted that immune deficiencies can be secondary to infections like HIV/AIDS or usage of drugs like corticosteroids; however, secondary immune deficiencies are beyond the scope of the discussion of this book.

Basic Components of the Immune System

Before discussing PIDs in-depth, let us quickly revise how the immune system functions to keep us healthy (Fig. 1.1):

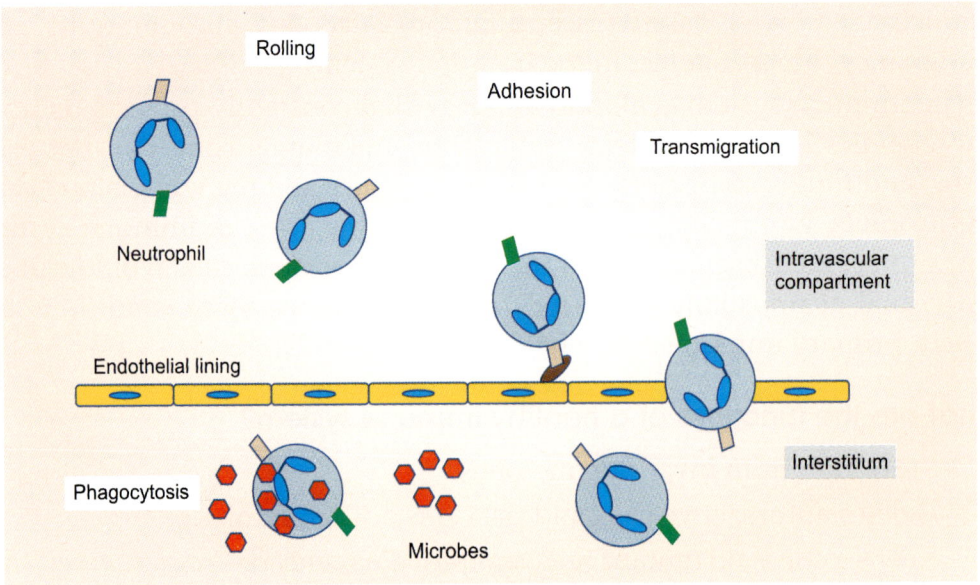

Fig. 1.1: Leukocyte adhesion and extravasation to the site of infection

A. When a microbe enters our body/tissue—tissue macrophages engulf the organism—*phagocytosis.*
B. Neutrophils present in the bloodstream leave the blood vessels to reach the tissues.

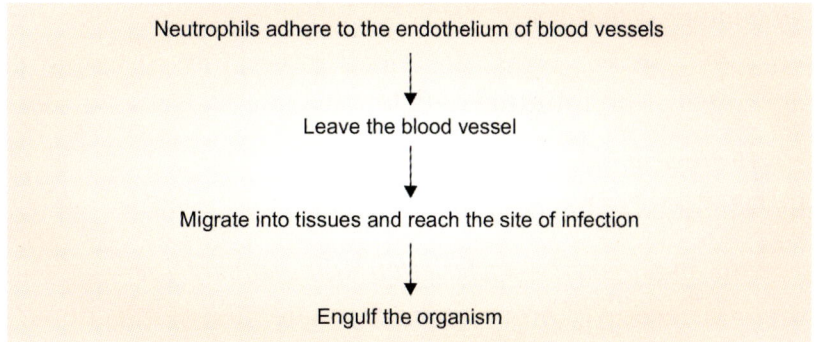

C. After phagocytosis, microbes are killed within macrophages and neutrophils. This process needs enzymes like NADPH oxidase.

Clinical implications

a. If neutrophils are absent in an individual, he/she would fail to handle pathogens (bacteria/fungi), e.g. severe congenital neutropenia.

b. If neutrophils cannot adhere to the endothelium, they would not be able to reach infected tissues. This would lead to recurrent infections, e.g. leukocyte adhesion deficiency.

c. If intracellular killing is defective, e.g. NADPH oxidase deficiency, this would lead to persistent infections and autoimmunity, e.g. chronic granulomatous disease.

T Cells and B Cells

a. B cells produce immunoglobulins (IgG, IgA, IgM and IgE) which handle various pathogens (predominantly extracellular bacteria). This is called *humoral (humor in greek meaning body fluid) immunity.*

b. T cells—CD8 T cells kill viral infected cells and play an important role in handling intracellular infections. This is called *cellular immunity.*

Clinical implications

1. Recurrent bacterial infections—think of B cell defect.
2. Viral/fungal infections—think of T cell defect.

Clinical Approach to Immune Deficiency

A systematic approach is needed to arrive to an appropriate diagnosis in a patient with suspected immune deficiency. One must attempt answering the following questions.

1. *Is it an immune deficiency?*
   Presence of warning signs (described in Chapter 3) would be strong pointer towards an immune deficiency.

2. *What is the type of immune defect?*
   B cell/combined/phagocytic/syndrome

3. *What are the organisms?—bacterial/viral/fungal/parasitic*
   Is it the same group of organisms causing recurrent infections? Or is the spectrum of infections very broad?

4. *Family history*—consanguinity, sibling deaths, recurrent infections in parents, issues in maternal uncles or male maternal cousins (X-linked inheritance).

5. Close look at all the previous **hemograms**. Calculate absolute neutrophil and lymphocyte counts (ANC and ALC).
   (congenital neutropenia, cyclic neutropenia can be diagnosed with hemograms.)

6. Look at the thymic shadow in chest radiograph in infants. (If absent, points towards severe combined immune deficiency).

7. Relevant immunological tests—immunoglobulins, lymphocyte subsets (T, B and NK cell counts), nitroblue tetrazolium test (NBT), dihydrorhodamine (DHR) assay.

8. Genetic testing.

9. Functional studies if indicated.

Did you know?

PIDs as a group are 4 times more common than hemophilia and 5 times more common than cystic fibrosis!

SUGGESTED READING

1. de Vries E; European Society for Immunodeficiencies (ESID) members. Patient-centred screening for primary immunodeficiency, a multi-stage diagnostic protocol designed for non-immunologists: 2011 update. *Clin Exp Immunol.* 2012; 167(1):108–119.

2. McCusker C, Upton J, Warrington R. Primary immunodeficiency. *Allergy Asthma Clin Immunol.* 2018 Sep 12; 14(Suppl 2):61.

3. Ochs HD, Hitzig WH. History of primary immunodeficiency diseases. *Curr Opin Allergy Clin Immunol.* 2012; 12(6):577–587.

Classification of Primary Immune Deficiency: What is clinically relevant?

> **The complete book of PID is yet to be written!**

The *International Union of Immunological Societies* (IUIS) publishes revised classification of primary immune deficiencies (PID), better known as inborn errors of immunity (IEI) every other year and the following article can be referred for the detailed classification.

Tangye SG, Al-Herz W, Bousfiha A, et al. Human Inborn Errors of Immunity: 2019 Update on the Classification from the International Union of Immunological Societies Expert Committee [published online ahead of print, 2020 Jan 17]. J Clin Immunol. 2020.

A phenotypic classification of inborn errors of immunity for practicing physicians and trainees can also be accessed at *Bousfiha A, Jeddane L, Picard C, et al. Human Inborn Errors of Immunity: 2019 Update of the IUIS Phenotypical Classification [published online ahead of print, 2020 Feb 11]. J Clin Immunol. 2020; 10.1007/s10875–020-00758-x. doi:10.1007/s10875–020-00758-x.*

Less than 100 PIDs were described back in 1999, and the following graph (Fig. 2.1) shows a tremendous surge in the numbers of newly diagnosed PIDs. The 2017 classification enlisted 354 diseases while the 2019 version has 416 inborn errors of immunity! Every year, several new diseases are being added to this rapidly expanding list, thanks to the phenomenal advancements in molecular science and next-generation sequencing (NGS) approaches. The latest IUIS classification provides 10 classes of IEIs (Table 2.1). However, as a clinician, when we face a child or an adult with recurrent/persistent/

unusual infection and an immune deficiency is suspected, we must attempt classifying them into one of the following four groups of PID (Fig. 2.2).

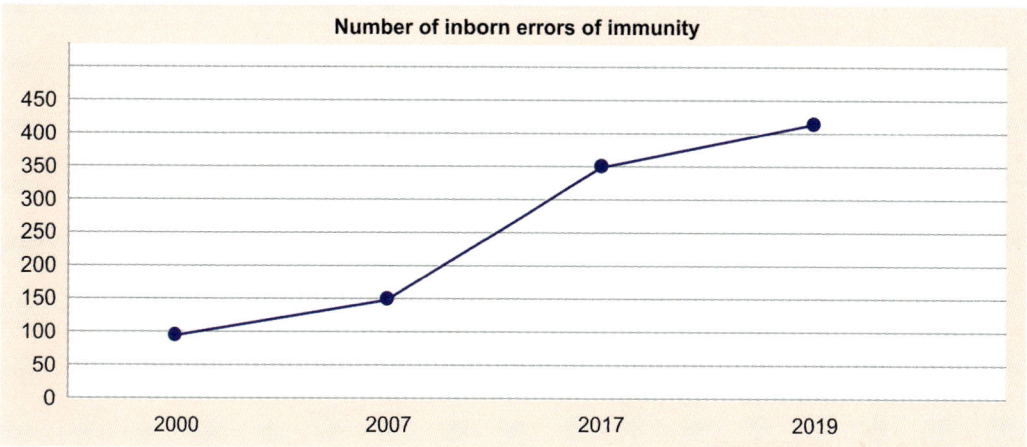

Fig. 2.1: Rising numbers of IEI over the past 2 decades

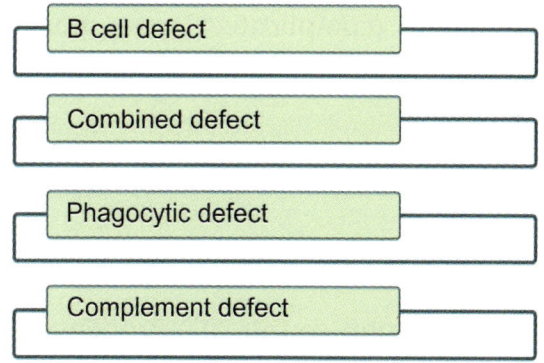

Fig. 2.2: Clinical classification of IEI

Salient clinical features that guide a clinician to classify a given patient into one of these groups are:

B Cell Defect

✦ Recurrent mucosal infections, e.g. recurrent sinusitis, recurrent pneumonia, recurrent diarrhea.

✦ Onset of symptoms beyond 6 months of age (as maternally transmitted IgG protects these infants during the first 6 months of life).

Evaluation suggested

+ Serum immunoglobulins and B cell counts.
+ Humoral or antibody response to vaccines (post-vaccination antibody titres).

T Cell/Combined Defect

+ Fungal and/or viral infections (e.g. *Aspergillus, Candida, Cytomegalovirus*) point towards an underlying cellular defect.
+ Severe forms of T cell defects have an onset in early infancy (e.g. severe combined immune deficiency).
+ Milder forms may have an onset later in life (e.g. combined immune defect due to LRBA deficiency, etc.).

Evaluation suggested

T cell counts (CD3 counts), serum immunoglobulins.

Phagocytic Defect

+ Suppurative infections (complicated pneumonia—empyema/lung abscess, hepatic abscess, suppurative lymphadenitis) are seen in phago-cytic defect.
+ Onset—severe forms present in infancy, while milder forms may present later in life.

Evaluation suggested

Look at the absolute neutrophil counts. Neutropenia may point towards severe congenital neutropenia/cyclic neutropenia. High neutrophil counts must make one think of chronic granulomatous disease (*nitroblue tetrazolium test and dihydrorhodamine test are the screening tests for chronic granulomatous disease*).

Complement Deficiency

+ Recurrent infections with encapsulated bacteria (*S. pneumoniae, H. influenzae*) can be noted in complement deficiency.
+ Early onset of autoimmune diseases can be a feature of complement deficiency (e.g. onset of lupus before the age of 5 years is seen in complement C1q deficiency).

✦ Individuals with recurrent infections with *Neisseria gonorrhoeae* or *Neisseria meningitidis* must be evaluated for terminal complement pathway defects (C5 to C9 deficiency).

Evaluation suggested

CH50 assay (functional assay for classical complement pathway), AP50 (functional assay for alternative pathway). If either or both of these assays is abnormal, individual complement components can be assessed based on clinical suspicion.

Note: A clinician dealing with a suspected case of PID must attempt classifying the index case into one of the above four major subclasses of PID. This would in turn lead to a targeted evaluation and early diagnosis, with the optimal utilization of the available diagnostic armamentarium.

Message: Pattern of infections, age at onset and type of organisms provide important clues to the underlying type of PID.

Table 2.1: 2019 IUIS classification of IEI
1. Immunodeficiencies affecting cellular and humoral immunity
2. Combined immunodeficiencies with associated or syndromic features
3. Predominantly antibody deficiencies
4. Diseases of immune dysregulation
5. Congenital defects of phagocyte number, function or both
6. Defects in intrinsic and innate immunity
7. Autoinflammatory diseases
8. Complement deficiencies
9. Bone marrow failure
10. Phenocopies of inborn errors of immunity

Did you know?

Phenocopies of PIDs are a special group of immune deficiencies.

+ They are not caused by a genomic mutation.
+ These are diseases wherein autoimmunity results in immune deficiency or there are somatic variants in PID genes!, e.g. anti-IL17 antibodies cause recurrent candidiasis.
+ They do not follow Mendelian pattern of inheritance.

SUGGESTED READING

1. Bousfiha A, Jeddane L, Picard C, et al. The 2017 IUIS Phenotypic Classification for Primary Immunodeficiencies. *J Clin Immunol*. 2018; 38(1):129–143.

2. Chapel H. Classification of primary immunodeficiency diseases by the International Union of Immunological Societies (IUIS) Expert Committee on Primary Immunodeficiency 2011. *Clin Exp Immunol*. 2012; 168(1):58–59.

3. Tangye SG, Al-Herz W, Bousfiha A, et al. Human Inborn Errors of Immunity: 2019 Update on the Classification from the International Union of Immunological Societies Expert Committee [published online ahead of print, 2020 Jan 17]. *J Clin Immunol*. 2020.

4. Singh A, Jindal AK, Joshi V, et al. An updated review on phenocopies of primary immunodeficiency diseases. *Genes Dis*. 2019; 7(1): 12–20.

Warning Signs of Immune Deficiency

> *Do not miss the forest for the trees!*

Popularly used warning signs of PID that have been valuable in raising awareness are listed in Table 3.1.

Table 3.1: Warning signs of PID

No.	Warning signs in children	Warning signs in adults
1.	Recurrent ear, nose, or throat infections; four or more new infections within 1 year	Recurrent ear, nose, or throat infections; two or more new infections within 1 year
2.	Two or more serious sinus infections within 1 year	Two or more serious sinus infections within 1 year
3.	Two or more pneumonias within 1 year	One pneumonia per year for more than 1 year
4.	Two or more months on antibiotics with no improvement or little effect	Recurrent viral infections (colds, herpes, warts, condyloma)
5.	Two or more deep-seated infections including septicemia	Infection with normally harmless tuberculosis-like bacteria
6.	Failure to thrive from early infancy	Chronic diarrhea with weight loss

Contd.

Table 3.1: Warning signs of PID (*Contd.*)

No.	*Warning signs in children*	*Warning signs in adults*
7.	Infection with atypical severity; recurrent pyogenic infections such as deep skin or organ abscesses	Infection with atypical severity; recurrent, deep abscesses of the skin or internal organs
8.	Infection with atypical pathogens; persistent thrush in mouth or fungal infections on skin	Infection with atypical pathogens; persistent thrush in mouth or fungal infections on skin
9.	Need for intravenous antibiotics to clear infections	Recurrent need for intravenous antibiotics to clear infections
10.	Family history of PID	Family history of PID

Presence of two or more warning signs warrants an evaluation for an underlying PID.

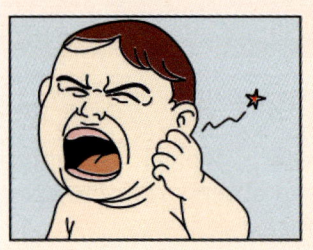

Four or more episodes of ear discharge

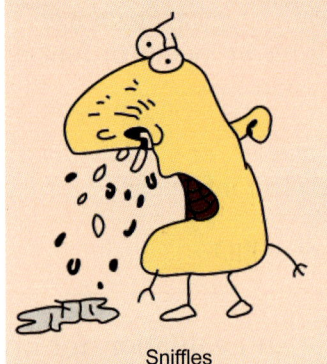

Sniffles

Two or more episodes of sinus infections within a year

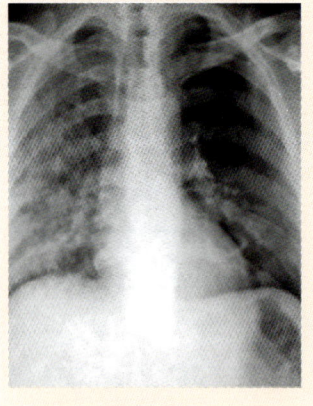

Two or more episodes of pneumonia

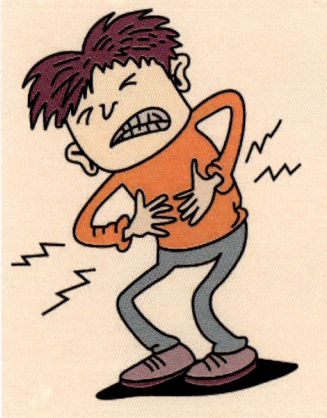

Repeated episodes of diarrhea

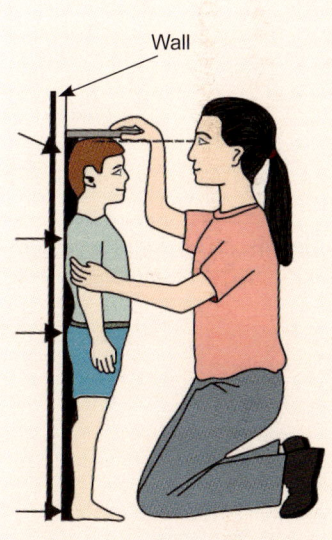

Wall

Failure to thrive—not gaining weight and height as per the age norms

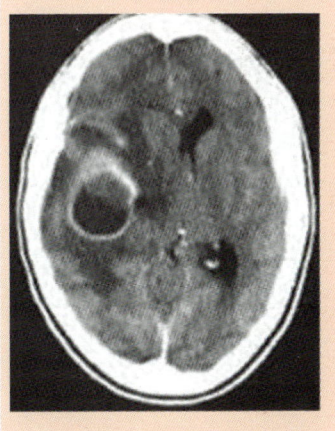

Repeated abscess formation (liver abscess, brain abscess)

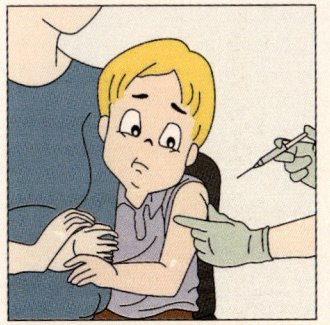

Infections warranting multiple hospitalizations

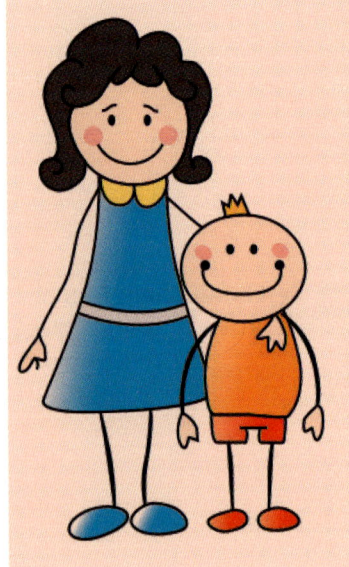

Family history of death of children at young age/due to immune deficiency

SUGGESTED READING

1. Arkwright PD, Gennery AR. Ten warning signs of primary immunodeficiency: a new paradigm is needed for the 21st century. *Ann N Y Acad Sci*. 2011; 1238:7–14.

2. Bjelac JA, Yonkof JR, Fernandez J. Differing Performance of the Warning Signs for Immunodeficiency in the Diagnosis of Pediatric Versus Adult Patients in a Two-Center Tertiary Referral Population. *J Clin Immunol*. 2019; 39(1):90–98.

3. Reda SM, El-Ghoneimy DH, Afifi HM. Clinical predictors of primary immunodeficiency diseases in children. *Allergy Asthma Immunol Res*. 2013; 5(2):88–95.

Rising Numbers of PID: Tip of the Iceberg!

First step to diagnose PID is TO THINK PID!

The number of cases diagnosed with PIDs is on the rise the world-over. Global report on the prevalence of PIDs published in 2011 (Jeffrey Modell Foundation—JMF network,[1] reported more than 60,000 patients with PID, while the latest report published in 2018[2] put this figure at around 1,80,000. This is the number of patients that have been reported by clinicians to JMF survey and is only the tip of the iceberg! The estimated prevalence of PID is 1 in 1200 cases and if we extrapolate this figure to the city of Bangalore, India, there must be around 5000 cases of PID in this city alone! But the actual number of cases diagnosed remains small.

These diseases are grossly under diagnosed and misdiagnosed. Patients often seek opinions from several doctors and hospitals. Many of them are hospitalized for several months and investigated extensively and yet fail to get an appropriate diagnosis. In severe forms of the disease (e.g. severe combined immune deficiency), families often would have lost many children before the index case gets diagnosed. These families suffer emotionally, financially and are often lost wandering from one hospital to another.

Over the last 3 years of my practice in Bangalore, we have diagnosed around 120 cases of PID. On average, 3 new cases per month! This is only the tip of the iceberg as awareness of these diseases at present in medical fraternity is minuscule. These diseases by no means are rare.

Another interesting finding in recent cohorts of PID published from the west is the exponential increase in the number of cases being diagnosed in adults. Around 60% of cases reported from the Jeffrey Modell Foundation

(JMF) network study (2011) were more than 18 years old! It is high time that adult physicians, pulmonologists and gastroenterologists start investigating unusual or unresolved cases for an underlying PID.

PIDs diagnosed at our centre* (including those referred from various hospitals) during 2017–2019 (Fig. 4.1).

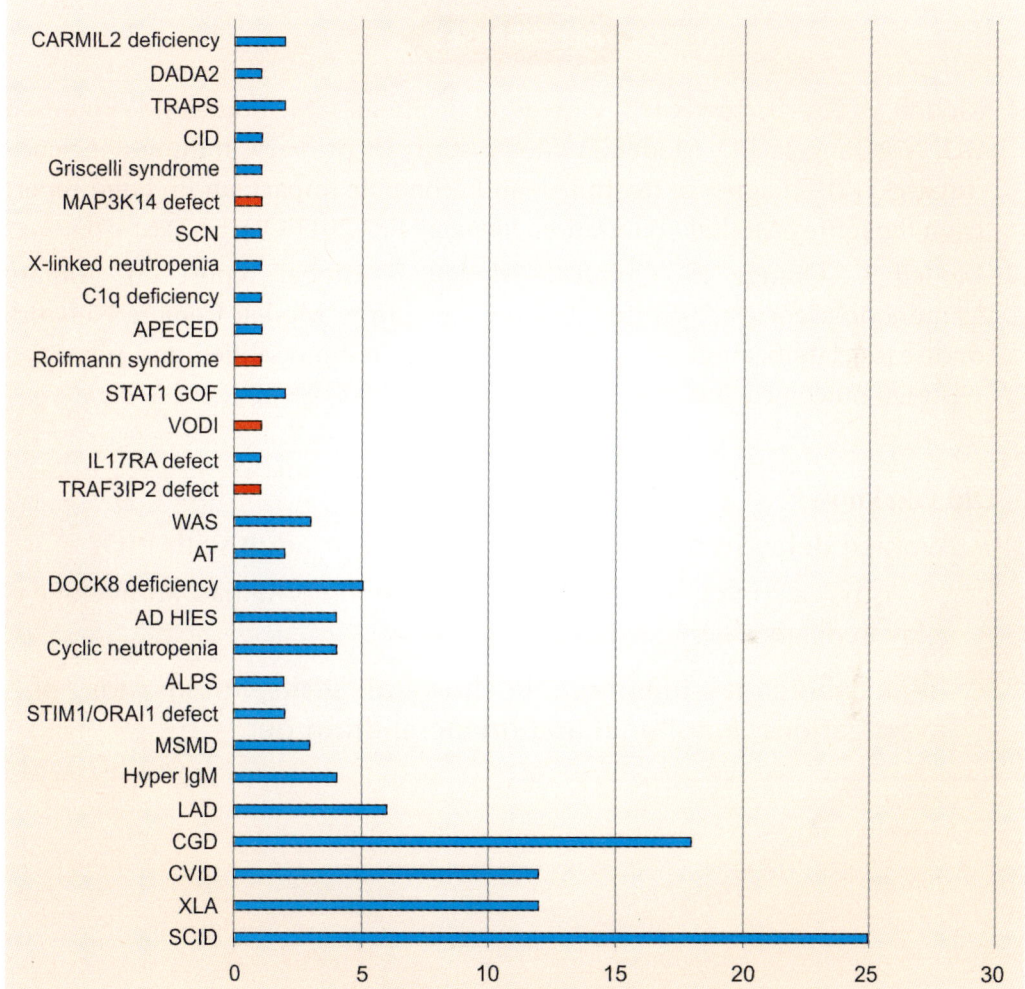

Fig. 4.1: Cases highlighted in red have been reported for the first time from the Indian subcontinent.

*Aster CMI Hospital, Bangalore, India.

(SCID—severe combined immune deficiency, XLA—X-lined agammaglobulinemia, CVID—common variable immunodeficiency, CGD—chronic granulomatous disease, LAD—leukocyte adhesion defect, MSMD—Mendelian susceptibility to mycobacterial disease, ALPS—autoimmune lymphoproliferative disease, AD HIES—autosomal dominant hyper IgE syndrome, AT—ataxia telangiectasia, WAS—Wiskott-Aldrich syndrome, VODI—veno-occlusive disease with immune deficiency, STAT1 GOF—STAT1 gain of function defect, APECED—autoimmune polyendocrinopathy candidiasis ectodermal dystrophy, SCN—severe congenital neutropenia, CID—combined immune defect, TRAPS—TNF receptor associated periodic fever syndrome, DADA2—deficiency of ADA2)

◀ REFERENCES ▶

1. Modell V, Gee B, Lewis DB, Orange JS, Roifman CM, Routes JM, Sorensen RU, Notarangelo LD, Modell F. Global study of primary immunodeficiency diseases (PI)—diagnosis, treatment, and economic impact: an updated report from the Jeffrey Modell Foundation. *Immunol Res.* 2011 Oct; 51(1):61–70.

2. Modell V, Orange JS, Quinn J, Modell F. Global report on primary immunodeficiencies: 2018 update from the Jeffrey Modell Centers Network ondisease classification, regional trends, treatment modalities, and physician reported outcomes. *Immunol Res.* 2018 Jun; 66(3):367–380.

Did you know?

✦ **Average delay in the diagnosis of a child or adult with PID?**

As per a survey in US (2007), adults with CVID had an average delay in diagnosis by 12.4 years!

✦ **Think about it—Innumerable hospital visits, thousands of investigations, emotional and financial drain-out.**

SUGGESTED READING

1. Jindal AK, Pilania RK, Rawat A, Singh S. Primary Immunodeficiency Disorders in India-A Situational Review. *Front Immunol.* 2017; 8:714.

2. Pilania RK, Chaudhary H, Jindal AK, et al. Current status and prospects of primary immunodeficiency diseases in Asia. Genes Dis. 2019; 7(1): 3–11.

3. Kobrynski L, Powell RW, Bowen S. Prevalence and morbidity of primary immunodeficiency diseases, United States 2001–2007. *J Clin Immunol.* 2014; 34(8):954–961.

Recurrent Pneumonia and Immune Deficiency

Pediatricians often evaluate children with recurrent pneumonia. Common differentials in this setting would be

a. Congenital heart disease (left to right shunts, ventricular septal defect)

b. Aspiration syndrome (e.g. gastroesophageal reflux disease)

c. Congenital lung malformation (e.g. congenital lobar emphysema)

d. Cystic fibrosis and ciliary dyskinesia

e. *Human immune deficiency virus* (HIV) infection

In all children and adults with recurrent pneumonia, primary immune deficiencies must be an important differential diagnosis.

Let us discuss this with few cases.

Case 1

A 3-year-old boy presented with fourth episode of pneumonia. He was hospitalized for 7–10 days during each of these episodes, treated with antimicrobials and received oxygen therapy. He was well in between these episodes.

He had been investigated extensively:

a. Echocardiography: Normal

b. Computed tomography (CT) chest: No anomaly

c. Sweat chloride test: Normal

d. Nuclear scan for GER: Normal (for gastro-esophageal reflux)

e. HIV rapid test: Non-reactive

He was referred to pediatric immunology services.

On a detailed clinical examination, tonsils were absent (Fig. 5.1). Lymph nodes were not palpable.

Note: Lymphoid growth is at its peak during 2–8 years of life.

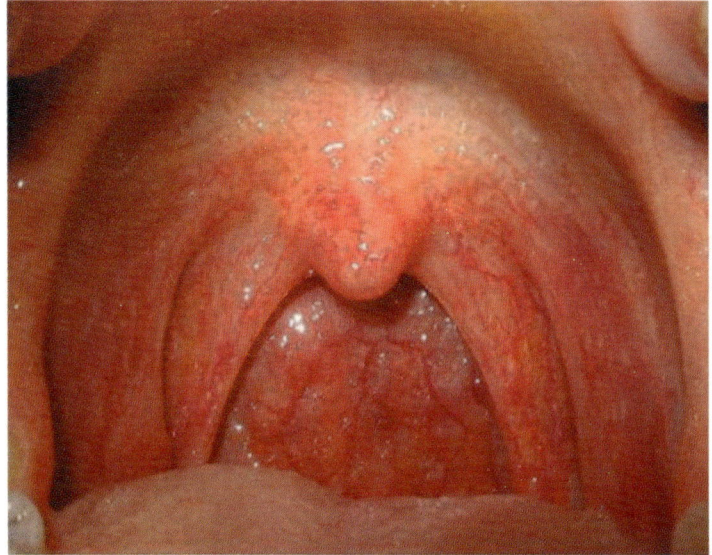

Fig. 5.1: Absent tonsils in a boy with X-linked agammaglobulinemia

Investigations

Complete blood count (CBC)—no neutropenia or lymphopenia.
He was investigated further.

Immunoglobulins:
+ IgG <130 mg/dl (345–1236)
+ IgA <30 mg/dl (14–159)
+ IgM <20 mg/dl (43–207)

All the immunoglobulins were low!

Next step: B cell counts were performed.
B cells (CD19): 0.5% (N 10–15%).

B cells were absent.

Database
3-year-old boy with recurrent pneumonia
↓
Absent tonsils and lymph nodes
↓
Low immunoglobulins and absent B cells
↓
Diagnosis: X-linked agammaglobulinemia

Message: Recurrent pneumonia—serum immunoglobulins must be tested.

A Quick Look into the Disease

X-linked Agammaglobulinemia (Previously called Brutons Agammaglobulinemia)

+ Boys are affected.
+ Recurrent pneumonia, otitis media, skin infections, diarrhea.
+ Absent tonsils.
+ Low immunoglobulins and absent B cells.
+ Mutation in the *BTK* gene.

Case 2

28-year-old gentleman was referred by the pulmonologist for immunological evaluation. He had had repeated episodes of pneumonia requiring 7–10 days of antimicrobials during each episode. He had 2–3 such episodes every year for the past 8 years.

Past History

Repeated episodes of ear discharge from the age of 10. Recurrent sinusitis from the age of 15–3 to four episodes/year (was said to have allergic rhinitis!).

He had been extensively evaluated before being referred.

CT chest done thrice revealed consolidation involving different lobes during these episodes of pneumonia. Latest CT chest showed changes of bronchiectasis in the lower lobes. He had undergone bronchoscopies but no definite diagnosis offered. He had been treated with antitubercular therapy twice empirically! HIV had been tested negative.

We looked at the immunoglobulin profile:
- ✦ IgG: 70 mg/dl (639–1349)
- ✦ IgA <26 mg/dl (70–312)
- ✦ IgM <20 mg/dl (56–352)

He had panhypogammaglobulinemia.

B cell counts: 15% (8–20%) {B cells were normal}

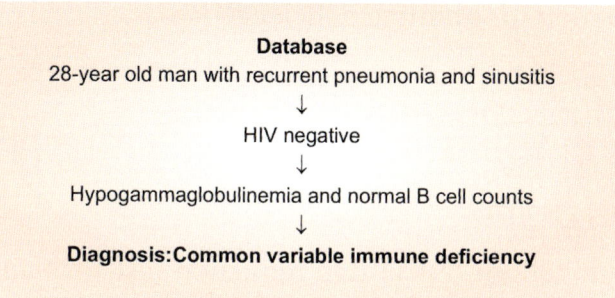

Database
28-year old man with recurrent pneumonia and sinusitis
↓
HIV negative
↓
Hypogammaglobulinemia and normal B cell counts
↓
Diagnosis:Common variable immune deficiency

Message: Recurrent pneumonia/rhinosinusitis in adults—look for immuno-globulins.

A Quick Look into the Disease

Common variable immune deficiency
- ✦ Commonest symptomatic immune deficiency (PID) seen in adults.
- ✦ Adolescents and adults present with recurrent pneumonia/recurrent sinusitis/recurrent or prolonged diarrhea/weight loss.
- ✦ Low immunoglobulins and normal B cells.
- ✦ *Grossly underdiagnosed in India!*
- ✦ *Immunoglobulin profile must be performed in patients with recurrent diarrhea and recurrent pneumonia.*
- ✦ *Gastroenterologists and pulmonologists must think of CVID while dealing patients with recurrent diarrhea and recurrent pneumonia, respectively.*

Persistent Pneumonia/Non-resolving Pneumonia

A 5-year-old child was hospitalized with severe pneumonia and was being ventilated. No improvement noted after 3 weeks of antibiotics (1st and 2nd line). Contrast enhanced CT (CECT) of the chest showed multiple nodules in lung parenchyma.

For definitive diagnosis, lung aspirate was performed and smears showed *Aspergillus*!

Diagnosis: *Aspergillus* pneumonia

Aspergillus is an unusual organism and infection with such organism(s) warrants evaluation for immune deficiency.

CBC: No neutropenia

IgG: 2300 mg/dl (345–1236),

IgA: 220 mg/dl (14–159),

IgM: 150 mg/dl (43–207).

Nitroblue tetrazolium (NBT) dye reduction test (explained in detail in Chapter 19) is a test to look for respiratory burst in neutrophils and is a screening test for chronic granulomatous disease (CGD). NBT was abnormal in the index case.

Diagnosis: Chronic granulomatous disease (CGD)

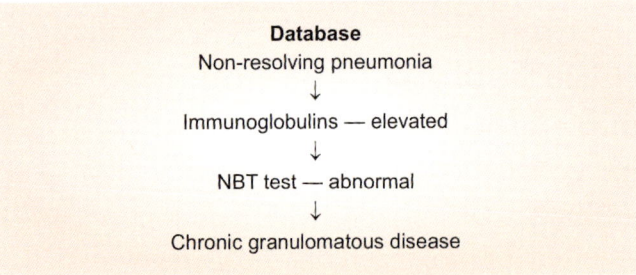

Database
Non-resolving pneumonia
↓
Immunoglobulins — elevated
↓
NBT test — abnormal
↓
Chronic granulomatous disease

Message
- A. Non-resolving pneumonia
  - i. Investigate for underlying organism
  - ii. Immune deficiency (phagocytic defect) likely

- B. *Aspergillus* pneumonia in non-neutropenic setting—always evaluate for CGD.

A Quick Look into the Disease

Chronic granulomatous disease

+ Defect in intracellular killing of engulfed organisms.
+ Phagocytic defect (defect in NADPH oxidase).
+ Suppurative infections—persistent pneumonia/lung abscess/liver abscess/lymphadenitis.
+ NBT and DHR—screening tests for diagnosis.

Did you know?

Dr Ogden Bruton described the first child with immune deficiency in 1952.

He noted absence of gamma globulins on recently described method of serum electrophoresis by Tiselius in a boy with recurrent pneumonia and treated him with subcutaneous injections of concentrated immune human globulin. This disease was later called X-linked agammaglobulinemia.

SUGGESTED READING

1. Jesenak M, Banovcin P, Jesenakova B, Babusikova E. Pulmonary manifestations of primary immunodeficiency disorders in children. *Front Pediatr*. 2014; 2:77.

2. Reisi M, Azizi G, Kiaee F, et al. Evaluation of pulmonary complications in patients with primary immunodeficiency disorders. *Eur Ann Allergy Clin Immunol*. 2017; 49(3):122–128.

3. Yazdani R, Abolhassani H, Asgardoon MH, et al. Infectious and Noninfectious Pulmonary Complications in Patients with Primary Immunodeficiency Disorders. *J Investig Allergol Clin Immunol*. 2017; 27(4):213–224.

Recurrent Otitis Media and Immune Deficiency

Repeated ear discharge (due to recurrent middle ear infections) can be a sign of underlying immune deficiency.

Case 1

A 2-year-old girl presented with repeated bilateral ear discharge from 3 months of life. She had been treated with antibiotics on multiple occasions. She also had repeated oral ulcers. She was now hospitalized with an episode of pneumonia.

CBC: Hb—10 g/dl, TC—7000/mm^3 (N$_3$, L$_{75}$, M$_{15}$, E$_6$, B$_1$), PC—230,000/mm^3

We must always look at the differential counts.
Absolute neutrophil count (ANC)—210/mm^3.

Note: ANC<1500 = Neutropenia; ANC<500 = Severe neutropenia

✦ Previous records were analysed and all of them showed ANC <1000.
✦ Bone marrow examination—maturation arrest in myeloid lineage (mature cells in myeloid lineage were absent).

Diagnosis: Severe congenital neutropenia

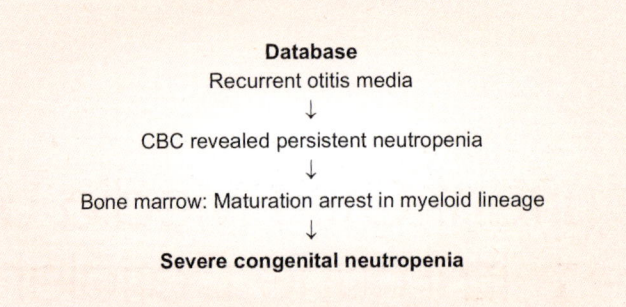

Database
Recurrent otitis media
↓
CBC revealed persistent neutropenia
↓
Bone marrow: Maturation arrest in myeloid lineage
↓
Severe congenital neutropenia

Case 2

6-year-old boy presented with multiple episodes of ear discharge from 3rd year of life.

At the age of 4, right sided mastoiditis. He developed seizures and was diagnosed to have meningitis. Received prolonged course of antibiotics and recovered.

At the age of 5, pneumonia.

In view of recurrent infections, he was referred to our department and was investigated.

HIV rapid card test: Negative

IgG <130 mg/dl,
IgA <30 mg/dl,
IgM <20 mg/dl.

B cells: Absent

Diagnosis: X-linked agammaglobulinemia

Message

1. Recurrent ear discharge can be a manifestation of PID
2. Differential counts provide very important clue to the underlying PID
3. One must look at serum immunoglobulins in patients with recurrent sino-pulmonary infections.

Did you know?

Kostmann disease was first described in 1956. This is a form of severe congenital neutropenia caused by mutation in HAX1 gene (AR inheritance).

SUGGESTED READING

1. Donadieu J, Beaupain B, Fenneteau O, Bellanné-Chantelot C. Congenital neutropenia in the era of genomics: classification, diagnosis, and natural history. *Br J Haematol*. 2017; 179(4):557–574.

2. Raje N, Dinakar C. Overview of Immunodeficiency Disorders. *Immunol Allergy Clin North Am*. 2015; 35(4):599–623.

Lung Abscess, Empyema, Liver Abscess, Suppurative Lymphadenitis

Children and adults who present with repeated suppurative lymphadenitis and/or deep seated abscesses (visceral abscess) must be evaluated for PID. These manifestations usually point to an underlying phagocytic defect.

Phagocytic Defect

A. Numerical defect → reduced number of neutrophils, e.g. severe congenital neutropenia, cyclic neutropenia

B. Functional defect → unable to kill intracellular organisms, e.g. chronic granulomatous disease

Let us look at few cases:

1. A 2-year-old boy presented with repeated infections and was referred for immunological evaluation.

   Review of history—

   ✦ 10 months of age: Fever and swelling of both feet. Radiographs of feet confirmed small bone *osteomyelitis* affecting multiple metatarsal bones (Fig. 7.1). Recovered after 2 months of intravenous antibiotics.
   ✦ 16 months of age: Blood in stools—treated for presumed dysentery.
   ✦ 18 months of age: Fever and right sided neck swelling—suppurative cervical *lymphadenitis*—pus was drained—culture—*Staphylococcus aureus*. He continued to have fever for a month despite being on appropriate antibiotics.

2. A 3-year-old boy admitted with severe necrotizing pneumonia. No response to broad spectrum antibiotics. CT scan of the chest during third week of illness revealed *lung abscess*.

3. A 6-year-old girl presented with fever and tender hepatomegaly. USG abdomen showed multiple *liver abscesses*. Pus was aspirated and culture grew *pseudomonas*.

4. A 7-year-old child presented with third episode of pneumonia. Chest radiograph showed pleural effusion. Pleural aspirate revealed frank pus. Diagnosed to have *empyema* and inter-coastal drainage (ICD) tube placed.

Would you investigate such cases for immune deficiency in day-to-day practice?

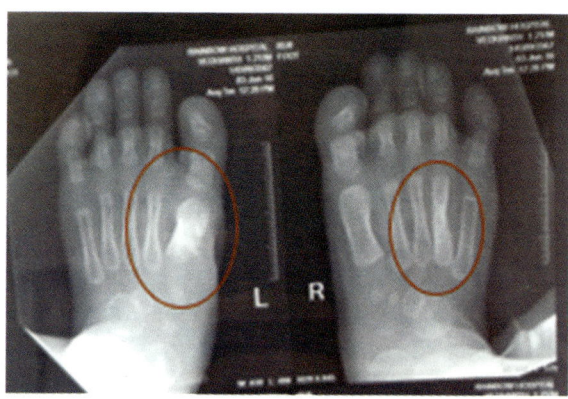

Fig. 7.1: Radiographs of the feet showing osteomyelitis affecting multiple metatarsal bones

Investigations in these cases				
	Case 1	Case 2	Case 3	Case 4
Hb (g/dl)	9	8.5	10	9.5
TC (per mm³)	20,000	18,000	15500	17300
DC	$N_{75}L_{15}$	$N_{70}L_{18}$	$N_{80}L_{16}$	$N_{78}L_{14}$
PC (per mm³)	600,000	650,000	800,000	550,000
IgG (mg/dl)	2100	1750	3200	1900
IgA (mg/dl)	150	220	345	180
IgM (mg/dl)	205	154	235	160

In all the above cases, marked neutrophilic leukocytosis was noted. Interestingly, platelet counts were high (500,000 to 800,000/mm³). Immunoglobulins were also elevated (*hypergammaglobulinemia*).

Nitroblue tetrazolium test and dihydrorhodamine tests were carried out. They were abnormal in all the cases.

Diagnosis: chronic granulomatous disease

Lessons learnt

1. Patients with suppurative infections (unusually severe or recurrent) and deep seated abscesses must be investigated. Phagocytic defect is likely in these settings.
2. Presence of normal or elevated immunoglobulins does not exclude immune deficiency. Hypergammaglobulinemia is a common feature in patients with CGD.
3. Marked leukocytosis and thrombocytosis may be seen in CGD.

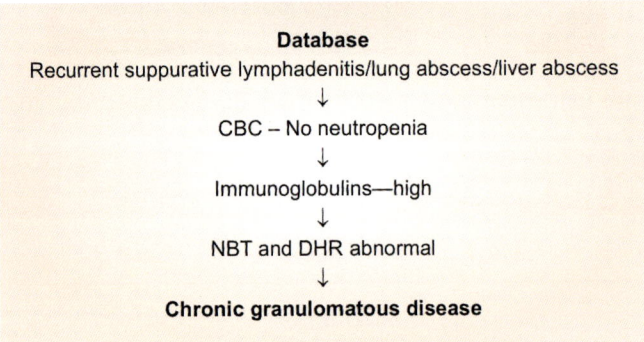

Database
Recurrent suppurative lymphadenitis/lung abscess/liver abscess
↓
CBC – No neutropenia
↓
Immunoglobulins—high
↓
NBT and DHR abnormal
↓
Chronic granulomatous disease

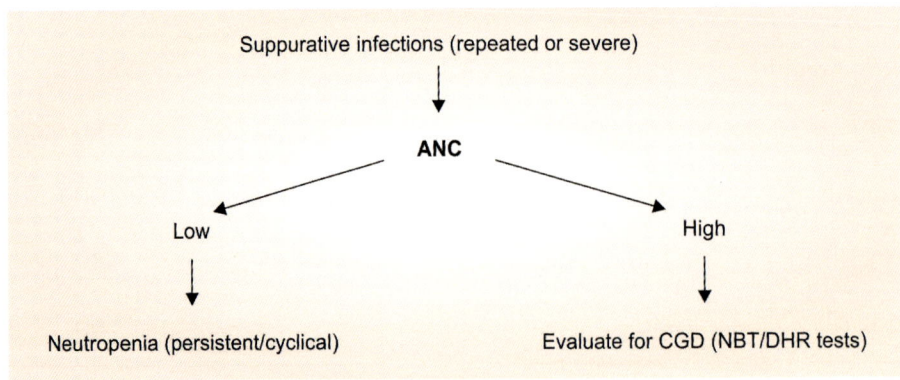

Suppurative infections (repeated or severe)
↓
ANC

Low → Neutropenia (persistent/cyclical)

High → Evaluate for CGD (NBT/DHR tests)

(ANC—absolute neutrophil count)

Did you know?

First case of chronic granulomatous disease was reported in 1954 with the following title.

"Hypergammaglobulinemia associated with severe, recurrent and chronic non-specific infection"

And the second case in 1957 as *"A fatal granulomatosus of childhood: The clinical study of a new syndrome"*

Both these case reports speak volumes of the characteristics of CGD—*hypergammaglobulinemia, granulomas, fatal*

SUGGESTED READING

1. Bennett N, Maglione PJ, Wright BL, Zerbe C. Infectious Complications in Patients With Chronic Granulomatous Disease. *J Pediatric Infect Dis Soc.* 2018 May 9; 7(suppl_1):S12–S17.

2. Rawat A, Bhattad S, Singh S. Chronic Granulomatous Disease. *Indian J Pediatr.* 2016; 83(4):345–353.

3. Rawat A, Vignesh P, Sharma A, et al. Infection Profile in Chronic Granulomatous Disease: a 23-Year Experience from a Tertiary Care Center in North India. *J Clin Immunol.* 2017; 37(3):319–328.

4. Yu JE, Azar AE, Chong HJ, Jongco AM 3rd, Prince BT. Considerations in the Diagnosis of Chronic Granulomatous Disease. *J Pediatric Infect Dis Soc.* 2018 May 9; 7(suppl_1):S6–S11.

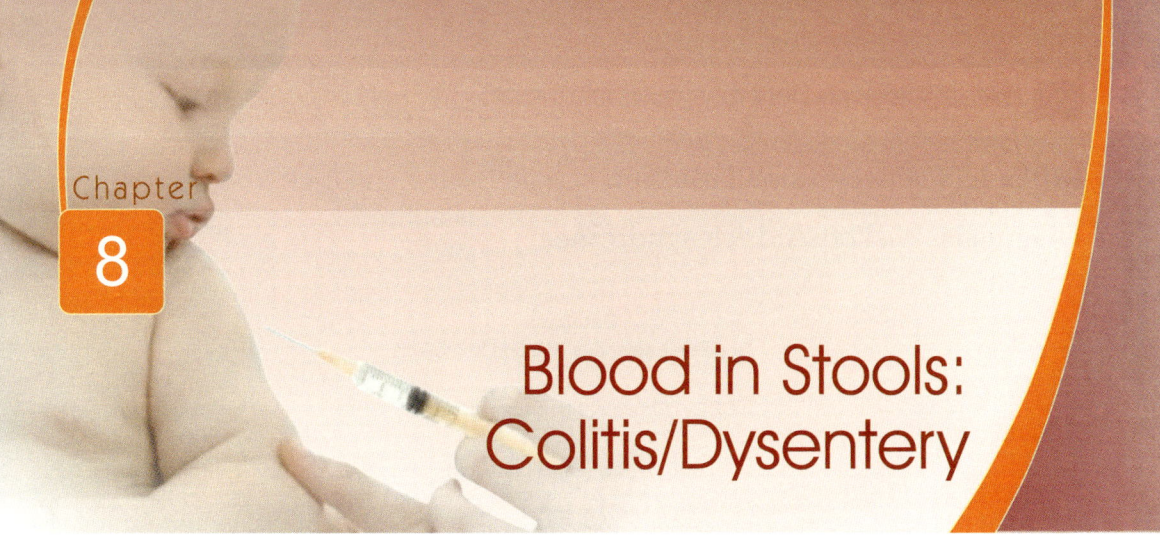

Blood in Stools: Colitis/Dysentery

During our clinical practice, we do come across children who develop fever, loose stools and blood in motions. These children are often diagnosed to have dysentery (bacterial/amoebic) and treated accordingly.

But have you come across cases in which children have repeated episodes of blood in motions? Are these children suffering from repeated episodes of dysentery?

Let us discuss few cases.

Case 1

A 2-year-old boy was admitted with pneumonia.

Past History

Three episodes of blood in motions from 6 months of age. Each time he had been treated with antibiotics (for suspicion of dysentery, though stool cultures were sterile).

Investigations

+ Hb: 10 g/dl
+ TC: 13000/mm^3 (N$_{55}$L$_{30}$E$_{10}$M$_5$)
+ PC: 30,000/mm^3

Thrombocytopenia was noted and was presumed to be caused by sepsis induced marrow suppression. But it was interesting to note *low platelet counts in all the previous records*!

We looked at the mean platelet volume (MPV).

MPV: 4.5 fl (7–11)→ small platelets

Diagnosis: Wiskott-Aldrich syndrome

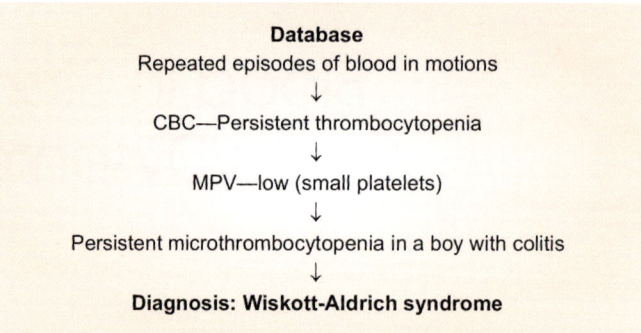

Message: In every child with persistent thrombocytopenia, one must look at MPV.

A Quick Look into the Disease

Wiskott-Aldrich syndrome

+ X-linked recessive inheritance
+ Recurrent infections + Eczema
+ Thrombocytopenia with small platelets
+ Recurrent blood in motions noted due to inflammatory colitis
+ Mutation in WASP gene

Case 2

A 3-year-old girl presented with repeated episodes of blood in motions for the past 2 years. She also had had 2 episodes of pneumonia, requiring inpatient treatment. She had been evaluated extensively for blood in motions. Colonoscopy and intestinal biopsies were non-rewarding (inflammatory bowel disease was excluded).

Investigations

+ CBC: Hb—9 g/dl, TC—20,000/mm^3 (N$_{70}$ L$_{20}$ M$_6$ E$_4$), PC—600,000/mm^3
+ ESR—120, CRP—80 mg/L (<6)

+ Blood and stool cultures: Sterile
+ HIV rapid card test: Negative

She was referred to the pediatric immunology services and was evaluated further.

IgG—2240 mg/dl (345–1236), IgA—190 mg/dl (14–159), IgM—280 mg/dl (43–207)

NBT and DHR tests were performed and were abnormal.

Diagnosis: Chronic granulomatous disease

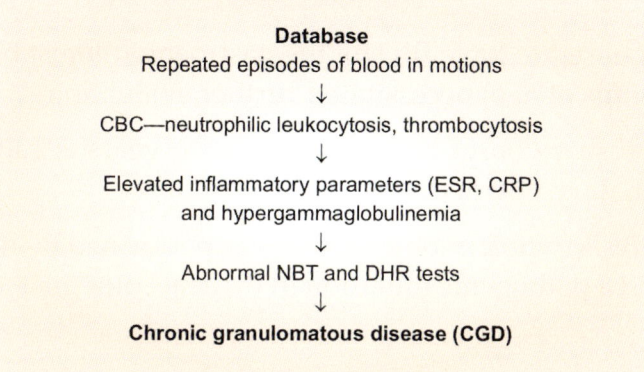

Database
Repeated episodes of blood in motions
↓
CBC—neutrophilic leukocytosis, thrombocytosis
↓
Elevated inflammatory parameters (ESR, CRP)
and hypergammaglobulinemia
↓
Abnormal NBT and DHR tests
↓
Chronic granulomatous disease (CGD)

Message: Recurrent blood in motions (colitis) is a known presentation in CGD.

Case 3

A 2.5-year-old boy born to a third degree consanguineously married couple, presented with repeated episodes of bloody diarrhea from 6 months of age. He would strain while passing stools and had tenesmus. At the age of one, he developed perianal abscess which was drained and treated with antibiotics. There was no history of recurrent ear infection, pneumonia or skin infections. He had significant failure to thrive (weight 9 kg, height 80 cm).

He was evaluated by the pediatric gastroenterologist and endoscopies (upper and lower GI) were performed.

Upper GI endoscopy: Normal

Lower GI endoscopy: Ulcers in the colonic mucosa.

Colonic biopsy: Cryptitis and crypt abscess suggestive of inflammatory bowel disease (IBD).

Further Evaluation

+ No thrombocytopenia (Wiskott-Aldrich syndrome was unlikely.)

+ HIV card test: Negative

+ Serum immunoglobulins were elevated.

+ NBT and DHR tests: Normal (CGD was excluded.)

He was diagnosed to have IBD by the gastroenterologist but early age of onset (at 6 months of age) necessitated further evaluation.

IBD with a disease onset before the age of 6 years is called **very early onset-inflammatory bowel disease (VEO-IBD).**

Genetic analysis (whole exome study) was performed by next generation sequencing and a pathogenic mutation in IL10 receptor gene was identified.

Diagnosis: VEO- IBD due to IL10R defect

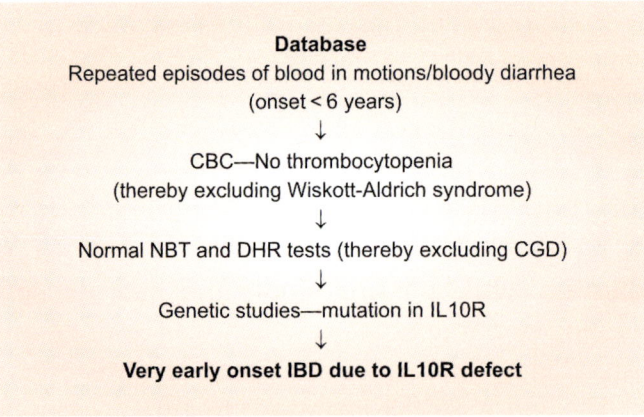

Database
Repeated episodes of blood in motions/bloody diarrhea
(onset < 6 years)
↓
CBC—No thrombocytopenia
(thereby excluding Wiskott-Aldrich syndrome)
↓
Normal NBT and DHR tests (thereby excluding CGD)
↓
Genetic studies—mutation in IL10R
↓
Very early onset IBD due to IL10R defect

Message: Onset of IBD at a very young age warrants evaluation for underlying genetic disease. Mutations in IL10 and IL10R genes can present with VEO-IBD.

A Quick Look into the Disease

VEO-IBD

+ Onset of IBD below 6 years of age.
+ Monogenic IBD.
+ Mutations in IL10 and IL10R genes.
+ Usually refractory to routinely used immunosuppressants.
+ Role for hematopoietic stem cell transplant.

Note: IL10 is an important anti-inflammatory cytokine and is critical for maintenance of immune homeostasis in gastro-intestinal tract.

Lessons Learnt

1. Recurrent blood in motions/bloody diarrhea can be the presenting feature of primary immune deficiency.
2. Recurrent bloody diarrhea + Thrombocytopenia in a boy = Wiskott-Aldrich syndrome
3. Recurrent bloody diarrhea = Evaluate for CGD
4. Very early onset IBD = Evaluate for IL10 and IL10R mutations.

Did you know?

Gastrointestinal tract (GIT) is the largest organ of the immune system. Secretory IgA plays an important role in immune tolerance, by trapping dietary antigens in the gut mucosa and prevents over-reaction of the immune system.

This may explain why patients with IgA deficiency have increased risk of allergies and autoimmune diseases!

SUGGESTED READING

1. Agarwal S, Cunningham-Rundles C. Gastrointestinal Manifestations and Complications of Primary Immunodeficiency Disorders. *Immunol Allergy Clin North Am.* 2019; 39(1):81–94.

2. Batura V, Muise AM. Very early onset IBD: Novel genetic aetiologies. *Curr Opin Allergy Clin Immunol.* 2018; 18(6):470–480.

3. Glocker E, Grimbacher B. Inflammatory bowel disease: Is it a primary immunodeficiency? *Cell Mol Life Sci.* 2012; 69(1):41–48.

4. Ohya T, Yanagimachi M, Iwasawa K, et al. Childhood-onset inflammatory bowel diseases associated with mutation of Wiskott-Aldrich syndrome protein gene. *World J Gastroenterol.* 2017; 23(48):8544–8552.

5. Shim JO. Recent Advance in Very Early Onset Inflammatory Bowel Disease. *Pediatr Gastroenterol Hepatol Nutr.* 2019; 22(1):41–49.

Recurrent Skin Infections and Eczema

When children and adults present with recurrent skin infections and/or chronic eczema, one must consider PID in the differential diagnosis. These patients are often seen by dermatologists and it would be prudent for dermatologists to be aware of PIDs to ensure a timely diagnosis in these patients.

Let us discuss few cases.

Case 1

A 15-year-old boy presented with recurrent skin infections/pyoderma from third year of life. He would develop cutaneous abscesses that warranted incision and drainage (I/D) of pus. He had undergone I/D procedures almost 7–8 times so far. He was also being treated with topical steroids for his chronic eczema. He presented to the pediatric department with fever, cough and rapid breathing. Chest radiograph showed consolidation and he was diagnosed to have pneumonia. Blood culture grew *Staphylococcus aureus*. He was treated with appropriate antibiotics.

Family background: Father also had had recurrent skin infections from his childhood. He also had pathological fracture involving bones of the right forearm after a trivial fall.

In view of the recurrent infections in the past, pediatric immunology consultation was sought.

Investigations

+ Hb—10 g/dl, TC—15000/mm^3 (N_{60} L_{20} M_8 E_{12}), PC—280,000/mm^3
+ HIV rapid card test: Negative
+ Immunoglobulins: IgG—1700 mg/dl, IgA—82 mg/dl, IgM—106 mg/dl
+ NBT and DHR: Normal

As the boy had been having chronic eczema, IgE levels were asked for.
+ IgE: 4240 U/L (N <60)
+ Father was also tested. IgE—3400 U/L (IgE was high)

Diagnosis: Hyper-IgE syndrome (AD)

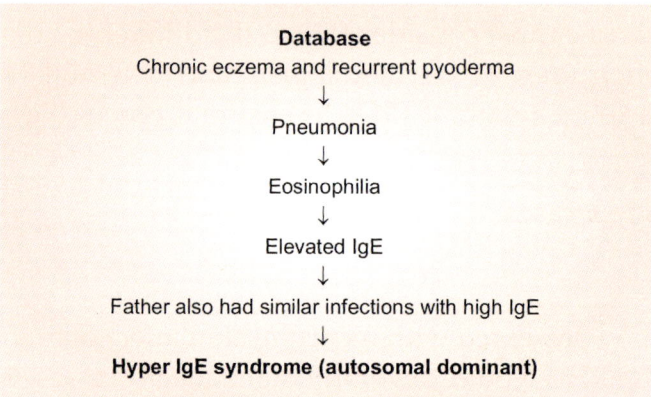

Database
Chronic eczema and recurrent pyoderma
↓
Pneumonia
↓
Eosinophilia
↓
Elevated IgE
↓
Father also had similar infections with high IgE
↓
Hyper IgE syndrome (autosomal dominant)

A Quick Look into the Disease

Hyper-IgE syndrome (AD)—Jobs syndrome

+ Children and adults present with recurrent skin infections, eczema and cold abscess (caused by *S. aureus*).
+ Coarse facial features which develop over time.
+ Delayed fall of primary dentition may be an important clue.
+ Pathological fractures.
+ Large pneumatoceles may be seen in chest radiograph.
+ **AD inheritance:** A detailed family history is very helpful.
+ Mutation in STAT3 gene.

> **Message:** In children and adults with recurrent skin infections, chronic eczema and high IgE levels, hyper-IgE syndrome must be considered as a differential.

Case 2

A 10-year-old boy presented with repeated skin infections and eczema. He had developed multiple warts all over the body and had extensive molluscum contangiosum.

Family history: Born to a consanguineously married couple and had lost 8-year-old girl sibling who had repeated skin and chest infections.

Investigations

+ HIV card test: Negative
+ CBC: Eosinophilia
+ IgE: 24,000 IU/ml (<60)

Genetic studies: Homozygous pathogenic mutation in DOCK8 gene

Diagnosis: Hyper-IgE syndrome (AR) due to DOCK8 defect

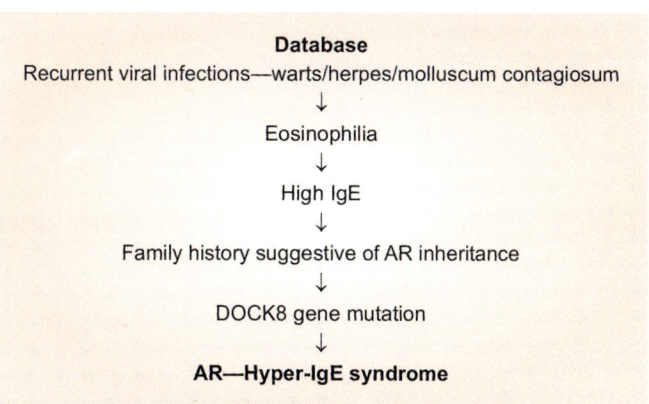

Database
Recurrent viral infections—warts/herpes/molluscum contagiosum
↓
Eosinophilia
↓
High IgE
↓
Family history suggestive of AR inheritance
↓
DOCK8 gene mutation
↓
AR—Hyper-IgE syndrome

> **Message:** Recurrent infections—extensive warts/herpes/molluscum contagiosum with very high IgE levels—look for mutation in DOCK8 gene.

Case 3

A 4-year-old boy presented with repeated pyoderma from first year of life. He had severe eczema and was being treated with topical steroids by the dermatologist. He was hospitalized with an episode of pneumonia.

Investigations

✦ CBC: Hb—10 g/dl, TC—13,000/mm^3 (N$_{65}$ L$_{20}$ M$_6$E$_9$), PC—60,000/mm^3
✦ HIV rapid card test: Negative

Please recall what we learnt in chapter 8.
In every child with persistent thrombocytopenia, one must look at MPV.

MPV: 5 fl (7–11) ⇒ This boy had microthrombocytopenia

Diagnosis: Wiskott-Aldrich syndrome

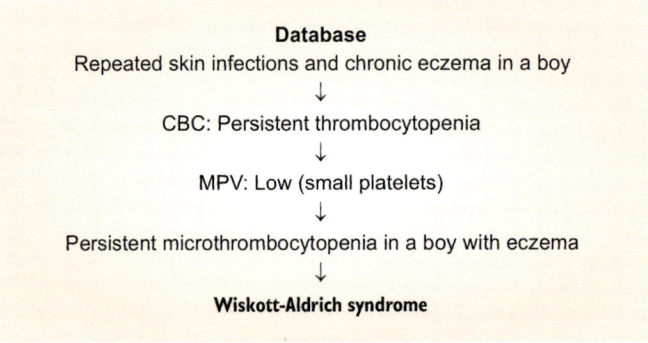

Database
Repeated skin infections and chronic eczema in a boy
↓
CBC: Persistent thrombocytopenia
↓
MPV: Low (small platelets)
↓
Persistent microthrombocytopenia in a boy with eczema
↓
Wiskott-Aldrich syndrome

Message: Chronic eczema + Low platelets = Wiskott-Aldrich syndrome

Lessons learnt

1. Eczema and recurrent skin infections can be a manifestation of underlying immune deficiency.
2. Autosomal dominant hyper-IgE syndrome (Jobs syndrome), autosomal recessive hyper-IgE syndrome (DOCK8 mutation), Wiskott-Aldrich syndrome are the differential diagnosis in this setting.
3. Presence of thrombocytopenia in boys with eczema is diagnostic of Wiskott-Aldrich syndrome; while children with extensive warts

and molluscum contangiosum must be evaluated for DOCK8 deficiency. Coarse facies with recurrent pyogenic infections and cold abscesses are pointers towards AD hyper-IgE syndrome (Jobs syndrome).

Did you know?

Cold skin abscess caused by *Staphylococcus* aureus is seen in patients with AD Hyper-IgE syndrome (Jobs syndrome).

SUGGESTED READING

1. Al-Herz W, Nanda A. Skin manifestations in primary immunodeficient children. *Pediatr Dermatol*. 2011; 28(5):494–501.

2. Lehman H, Gordon C. The Skin as a Window into Primary Immune Deficiency Diseases: Atopic Dermatitis and Chronic Mucocutaneous Candidiasis. *J Allergy Clin Immunol Pract*. 2019; 7(3):788–798.

3. Minegishi Y, Saito M. Cutaneous manifestations of Hyper-IgE syndrome. *Allergol Int*. 2012; 61(2):191–196.

4. Moin A, Farhoudi A, Moin M, Pourpak Z, Bazargan N. Cutaneous manifestations of primary immunodeficiency diseases in children. *Iran J Allergy Asthma Immunol*. 2006; 5(3):121–126.

5. Sillevis Smitt JH, Kuijpers TW. Cutaneous manifestations of primary immunodeficiency. *Curr Opin Pediatr*. 2013; 25(4):492–497.

Disseminated BCG Infection and Immune Deficiency

BCG vaccine is routinely administered to all babies at birth in India and most of the developing world. BCG is a live attenuated vaccine. Localized adenitis (left axillary) is known to occur in a small subset of healthy children and does not warrant any immunological evaluation. However, the presence of disseminated BCG infection must be investigated, as dissemination of attenuated bacteria indicates an underlying immunological defect.

Case 1

A 3-month-old girl child presented with fever, generalized lymphadenopathy and hepatosplenomegaly. Aspiration of the right axillary node showed acid-fast bacilli, which was confirmed to be BCG by culture.

Diagnosis: Disseminated BCG infection.

Investigations

CBC showed persistent lymphopenia (ALC <3000/mm^3).
   Further evaluation,
   + IgG <130 mg/dl
   + IgA <17 mg/dl
   + IgM <15 mg/dl

Lymphocyte subsets: T—0.5% B—95% NK—1%(T-B+NK-)
Infants with lymphopenia + Low T cells + Hypogammaglobulinemia = Severe combined immune deficiency (SCID)

Diagnosis: Severe combined immune deficiency with disseminated BCG infection.

Case 2

A 7-month-old boy presented with fever for 1 month. Past history was significant. He had been having rashes over scalp and trunk from first month of life. He had been hospitalized and treated for pneumonia at the age of 1 month. Examination showed generalized lymphadenopathy and hepatosplenomegaly.

Investigations

CBC: Hb—9 mg/dl, TC—17000/mm^3 (N_{70} L_{25} M_3 E_2), PC—9,20,000/mm^3 {Marked thrombocytosis and neutrophilic leukocytosis; no lymphopenia}. Right cervical node biopsy showed caseating granuloma, acid-fast bacilli ++, culture: BCG strain.

Diagnosis: Disseminated BCG infection

Immunological work-up:
+ IgG—1100 mg/dl (172–1069)
+ IgA—180 mg/dl (11–106)
+ IgM—230 mg/dl (33–126) {hypergammaglobulinemia noted}
+ **NBT and DHR tests: Abnormal**

Final diagnosis: Chronic granulomatous disease (CGD) with disseminated BCG infection.

Case 3

A 6-month-old girl presented with fever and generalized lymphadenopathy. BCG site was ulcerated (Fig. 10.1). On evaluation, she was diagnosed to have disseminated BCG infection.

Further work-up

+ Immunoglobulins: Normal
+ Lymphocyte subsets (T, B, NK cells): Normal
+ NBT and DHR tests: Normal

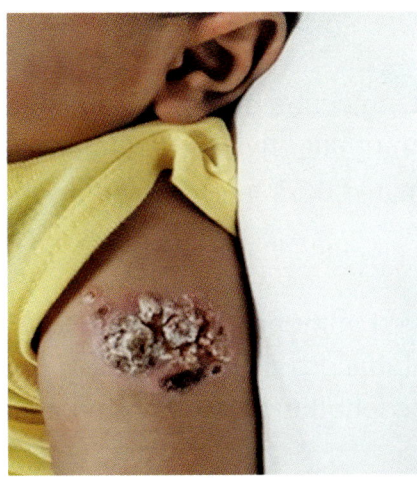

Fig. 10.1: Ulcerated BCG vaccination site in a 6-month old child.

Genetic studies: Homozygous mutation in IL12Rß1 gene, confirming Mendelian susceptibility to mycobacterial disease (MSMD).

Diagnosis: Mendelian susceptibility to mycobacterial disease (MSMD) due to IL12Rß1deficiency, with disseminated BCG infection.

Treatment: She was started on antitubercular therapy (isoniazid, rifampicin, ethambutol and levofloxacin; which was given for the next 2 years). Currently, the child is 4-year-old and is doing fine.

Note: BCG is inherently resistant to pyrazinamide.

A Quick Look into the Disease

Mendelian susceptibility to mycobacterial disease (MSMD)

+ Group of rare genetic disorders.
+ Defect in interferon γ (IFN γ)—mediated immunity. Also known as IL12/IL23-IFN γ pathway defects.
+ Infections with atypical and low virulent mycobacteria, like the Bacillus Calmette-Guèrin (BCG) vaccines and the non-tubercular environmental mycobacteria.
+ Genetic studies—mutation in IL12Rβ1, IFN γR1, IFN γR2 etc.
+ Severe forms need bone marrow transplant.

Message

1. Disseminated BCG infection or infections with atypical mycobacteria warrant evaluation for underlying immune defect.

2. In case of disseminated BCG infection, following differentials must be considered:

   a. HIV infection
   b. Severe combined immune deficiency (SCID)
   c. Chronic granulomatous disease (CGD)
   d. Mendelian susceptibility to mycobacterial disease (MSMD)

Did you know?

IL-12 secretion has a crucial role in host defence against mycobacteria. Its critical role resides in the induction of IFN-γ production by T cells and represents the junction between innate and adaptive immunity.

SUGGESTED READING

1. Al-Hammadi S, Alsuwaidi AR, Alshamsi ET, Ghatasheh GA, Souid AK. Disseminated Bacillus Calmette-Guérin (BCG) infections in infants with immunodeficiency. *BMC Res Notes*. 2017; 10(1):177.

2. Bhattad S. Mendelian Susceptibility to Mycobacterial Disease: A Clinical and Laboratory Approach. *Ped Inf Dis.*2019; 1 (1): 34–36.

3. Bustamante J, Boisson-Dupuis S, Abel L, Casanova JL. Mendelian susceptibility to mycobacterial disease: genetic, immunological, and clinical features of inborn errors of IFN- immunity. *Semin Immunol*. 2014; 26(6):454–470.

4. Reed B, Dolen WK. The Child with Recurrent Mycobacterial Disease. *Curr Allergy Asthma Rep*. 2018; 18(8):44.

5. Rosain J, Kong XF, Martinez-Barricarte R, et al. Mendelian susceptibility to mycobacterial disease: 2014–2018 update. *Immunol Cell Biol*. 2019; 97(4): 360–367.

Recurrent Candidiasis and Immune Deficiency

Candidiasis is an opportunistic infection and individuals presenting with recurrent or persistent candidiasis must be investigated for underlying PID. It is essential to note that T cells and neutrophils are essential to eliminate candida in a healthy individual. Recurrent candidiasis can thus be noted in T cell and phagocytic defects. Th17 cells (a type to T helper cell) play pivotal role in handling candida and children presenting with predominant susceptibility to candida must be evaluated for Th17 pathway defects.

Let us discuss few cases.

Case 1

A 5-month-old girl presented with recurrent episodes of oral thrush from first month of life. She had been treated with topical antifungals by the pediatrician. A course of oral fluconazole had also been prescribed. She had an episode of pneumonia at 3 months of age, that responded to intravenous antibiotics. In view of persistent thrush, she was referred to pediatric immunology services.

Investigations

✦ HIV rapid test: Negative
✦ CBC: Hb—8.8 mg/dl, TC—11,000/mm^3 (N$_{84}$L$_6$ M$_6$ E$_4$), PC—143,000/mm^3
✦ ANC: 9240, ALC:660 (lymphopenia noted)

Immunological Work-up

+ IgG <130 mg/dl
+ IgA <17 mg/dl
+ IgM <15 mg/dl
+ Lymphocyte subsets: T—1% B—98% NK—1% (T-B+NK-)
  Low immunoglobulins and absent T cells

Diagnosis: Severe combined immune deficiency

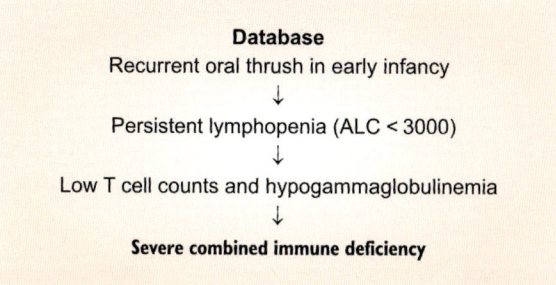

Database
Recurrent oral thrush in early infancy
↓
Persistent lymphopenia (ALC < 3000)
↓
Low T cell counts and hypogammaglobulinemia
↓
Severe combined immune deficiency

Case 2

A 7-year-old boy presented with recurrent episodes of skin infections (pyoderma) from 2 years of age. He had been treated with IV antibiotics for orbital abscess at the age of 6. On further enquiry, parents reported recurrent episodes of oral thrush from the age of 3. He had received multiple courses of oral fluconazole for the same. Thrush would improve on therapy, only to recur, once antifungals were stopped.

On examination, nails showed onychomycosis (Fig. 11.1).

Evaluation

+ Hemogram showed eosinophilia.
+ HIV rapid card test: Negative

Immunoglobulins

+ IgG: 1100 mg/dl (608–1572)
+ IgA: 86 (33–236)
+ IgM: 115 (43–207)
+ IgE: 2300 IU (N <60) {IgE was markedly elevated}

Genetic studies: Mutation in STAT3 gene

Diagnosis: Hyper-IgE syndrome (AD)

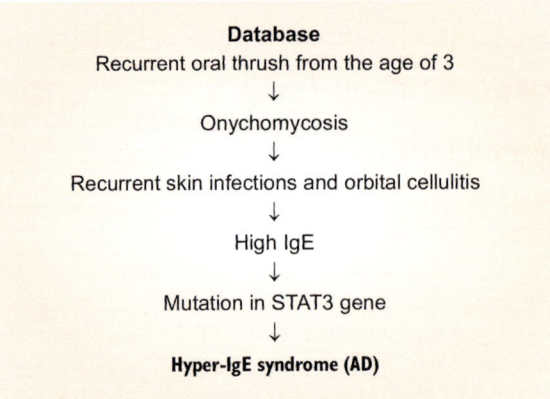

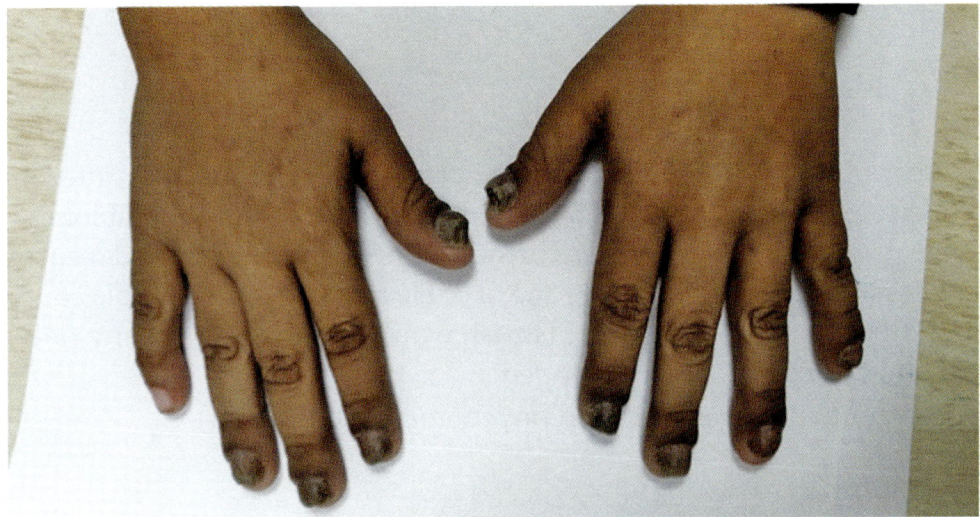

Fig. 11.1: Onychomycosis in a child with AD hyper-IgE syndrome.

Case 3

A 1-year-old girl presented with repeated episodes of oral thrush from 3 months of age. She also had been treated for disseminated CMV infection (pneumonia/hepatitis/colitis) at the age of 6 months. In view of severe CMV infection and recurrent candidiasis, she was suspected to have an immune deficiency and referred to our department.

Investigations

- HIV card test: Negative
- CBC: Normal (no neutropenia or lymphopenia)
- Immunoglobulins: Within normal limits
- Lymphocyte subsets (CD3, CD19, CD56, CD4 and CD8)—Normal

As the suspicion of immune deficiency was high on cards, we proceeded with the genetic testing.

Genetic studies (whole exome sequencing by NGS): Heterozygous mutation in STAT1 gene, suggestive of gain of function defect in STAT1 gene

Final diagnosis: STAT1 gain of function defect causing chronic mucocutaneous candidiasis (CMC) syndrome.

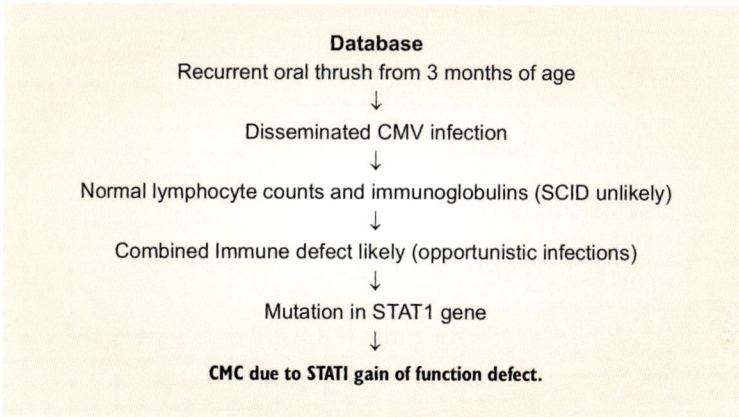

Database
Recurrent oral thrush from 3 months of age
↓
Disseminated CMV infection
↓
Normal lymphocyte counts and immunoglobulins (SCID unlikely)
↓
Combined Immune defect likely (opportunistic infections)
↓
Mutation in STAT1 gene
↓
CMC due to STATI gain of function defect.

Chronic Mucocutaneous Candidiasis (CMC)

+ A group of disorders characterised by increased susceptibility to candidiasis.
+ Defect in Th17 pathway is noted in most of them.
+ Present with oropharyngeal candidiasis and/or onychomycosis.
+ May be susceptible to other organisms (e.g. *S. aureus*) based on the underlying genetic defect.

CMC can be seen in the following diseases.

AD hyper-IgE syndrome (STAT3 deficiency)
STAT1 gain of function defect
CARD9 deficiency
IL17RA deficiency
IL17F deficiency
TRAPF3IP2 deficiency
APECED (*AIRE* mutation)
AR hyper-IgE syndrome (DOCK8 deficiency)

Message
1. Recurrent or persistent candidiasis is an indicator of underlying immune defect.
2. Recurrent candidiasis + lymphopenia in infancy »»» Severe combined immune deficiency (SCiD)
3. Mucocutaneous candidiasis »»» Defect in Th17 cells or IL17 signaling defects.

Did you know?
While patients with Th17 defects develop mucocutaneous candidiasis, those with neutropenia develop invasive fungal infection.

SUGGESTED READING

1. Bhattad S, Dinakar C, Pinnamaraju H, Ganapathy A, Mannan A. Chronic Mucocutaneous Candidiasis in an Adolescent Boy Due to a Novel Mutation in TRAF3IP2. *J Clin Immunol.* 2019; 39(6):596–599.

2. Lanternier F, Cypowyj S, Picard C, et al. Primary immunodeficiencies underlying fungal infections. *Curr Opin Pediatr.* 2013; 25(6):736–747.

3. Pichard DC, Freeman AF, Cowen EW. Primary immunodeficiency update: Part II. Syndromes associated with mucocutaneous candidiasis and noninfectious cutaneous manifestations. *J Am Acad Dermatol.* 2015; 73(3):367–382.

4. Antachopoulos C, Walsh TJ, Roilides E. Fungal infections in primary immunodeficiencies. *Eur J Pediatr.* 2007; 166(11):1099–1117.

5. Carey B, Lambourne J, Porter S, Hodgson T. Chronic mucocutaneous candidiasis due to gain-of-function mutation in STAT1. *Oral Dis.* 2019; 25(3):684–692.

6. Lilic D. New perspectives on the immunology of chronic mucocutaneous candidiasis. *Curr Opin Infect Dis.* 2002; 15(2):143–147.

7. Veverka KK, Feldman SR. Chronic mucocutaneous candidiasis: what can we conclude about IL-17 antagonism? *J Dermatolog Treat.* 2018; 29(5):475–480.

Autoimmunity and Immune Deficiency

It may be surprising to know that children and adults with primary immune deficiency can present with autoimmune manifestations.

How can an immune system that cannot efficiently tackle pathogens, have an ability to attack one's own tissues? Isn't it paradoxical?

Let us revise what we learnt in the 'Introduction Chapter'.

Functions of a healthy immune system include:

1. Protect oneself from infections
2. Delete autoreactive cells and prevent autoimmunity
3. Keep a check on mutant cells and prevent cancers: Cancer surveillance

Thereby, a defective immune system predisposes to autoimmunity.

Let me present a few relevant cases.

Case 1

A 28-year-old lady presented with repeated episodes of pneumonia from 5 years of age. She also had had multiple episodes of sinusitis and ear infections. She had arthritis affecting small joints of the hands and feet along with elbows, wrists and knees from the age of 12 and was being treated for 'juvenile idiopathic arthritis' with NSAIDs and methotrexate.

As she continued to have episodes of pneumonia, she was referred to the Immunology services for evaluation.

Investigations

+ HIV card test: Negative
+ IgG: 220 mg/dl (639–1349)

+ IgA: 42 mg/dl (70–312)
+ IgM: 50 mg/dl (56–352)

B cell counts: 12% (8–20%) {B cells were normal}

Diagnosis: Common variable immune deficiency

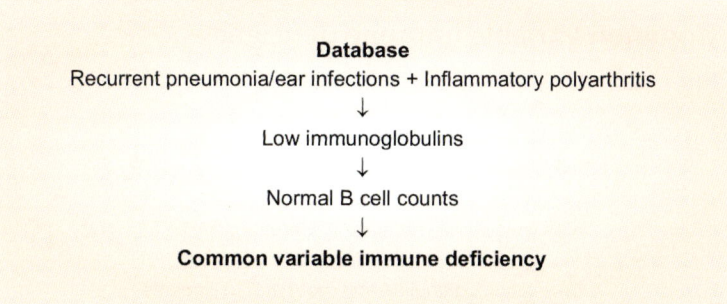

Database
Recurrent pneumonia/ear infections + Inflammatory polyarthritis
↓
Low immunoglobulins
↓
Normal B cell counts
↓
Common variable immune deficiency

Message
1. **Arthritis is a well-known manifestation of PID.**
2. **Arthritis + Recurrent infections = Serum immunoglobulins must be looked into.**

Case 2

A 25-year-old female presented with malar rash over cheeks (butterfly rash), oral ulcers, alopecia and arthritis. She was thought to have systemic lupus erythematosus (SLE). Past history was significant. She had purpuric rashes at the age of 5 and was diagnosed to have ITP (immune thrombocytopenic purpura). Her platelet counts were 30,000/mm³. She had received steroids for chronic ITP. Her platelets had normalized by the age of 10.

Evaluation for suspected SLE

+ ANA (antinuclear antibody test): Negative
+ Anti-dsDNA: Negative
+ Complements C3 and C4 were low.
+ ESR: 120 mm/1st hr

Low complements in the background of malar rash, oral ulcers, alopecia and arthritis strongly pointed towards a diagnosis of SLE, but a negative ANA remained unexplained!

On further evaluation:

+ IgG <200 (639–1349)
+ IgA: 35 (70–312)
+ IgM: 27 (56–352)

B cell counts were normal.

Diagnosis: Common variable immune deficiency

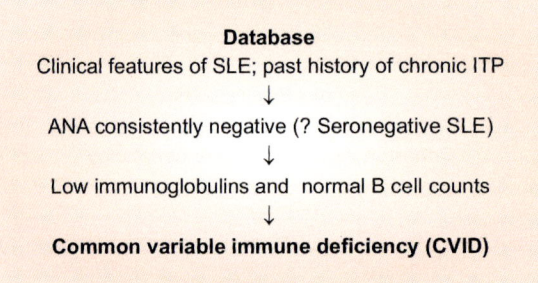

Database

Clinical features of SLE; past history of chronic ITP
↓
ANA consistently negative (? Seronegative SLE)
↓
Low immunoglobulins and normal B cell counts
↓
Common variable immune deficiency (CVID)

Message: Autoimmune cytopenia/lupus can be noted in patients with CVID.

Case 3

A 3-year-old boy presented with malar rash, diffuse alopecia and oral ulcers for the past 1 year.

Evaluation: ANA 4 + (strongly positive)
ANA profile: Anti-Sm ++, anti-Ro ++

Diagnosis: Systemic lupus erythematosus.

This child had onset of SLE at the age of 2!

SLE is most commonly noted in young females and childhood SLE usually starts after the age of 10. Onset of SLE below the age of 5 is extremely uncommon. Further evaluation was considered necessary. Serum C1q levels and CH50 assay were performed. Both were markedly reduced.

Genetic studies: Homozygous pathogenic mutation in C1QA gene.

Diagnosis: Complement C1q deficiency (presenting with early onset SLE).

> **Database**
> Onset of SLE at the age of 2
> ↓
> ANA strongly positive, anti-Sm positive
> ↓
> Low CH50, reduced C1q levels
> ↓
> Mutation in C1QA gene
> ↓
> **Complement C1q deficiency**

Message: Early onset SLE (below the age of 5): Evaluate for underlying complement deficiency.

Note: C1q is the first complement protein in the classical complement pathway, which is activated by antigen–antibody complex. Absence of C1q leads to failure of activation of this pathway.

C1q—clears immune complex. Deficiency of C1q leads to accumulation and deposition of immune complexes in the tissues → autoimmunity.

Lessons learnt

1. Autoimmunity (arthritis, autoimmune cytopenia, SLE, etc.) are well-known in patients with PID.
2. Arthritis + Recurrent infections → Evaluate for PID (immunoglobulins must be looked into)
3. Early onset autoimmunity → Evaluate for PID.

   Early onset SLE can be monogenic lupus. Evaluate for underlying complement deficiency in children with onset of SLE below the age of 5.

Did you know?

+ Complement C1q is produced by monocyte/macrophages, immature dendritic cells and mast cells, while other complement proteins are produced in the liver.
+ Patients with C1q deficiency can thus be cured with a bone marrow transplant!

SUGGESTED READING

1. Azizi G, Ziaee V, Tavakol M, et al. Approach to the Management of Auto-immunity in Primary Immunodeficiency. *Scand J Immunol*. 2017; 85(1):13–29.

2. Bhattad S, Rawat A, Gupta A, et al. Early Complement Component Deficiency in a Single-Centre Cohort of Pediatric Onset Lupus. *J Clin Immunol*. 2015; 35(8):777–785.

3. Dimitriades VR, Sorensen R. Rheumatologic manifestations of primary immunodeficiency diseases. *Clin Rheumatol*. 2016; 35(4):843–850.

4. Lehman HK. Autoimmunity and Immune Dysregulation in Primary Immune Deficiency Disorders. *Curr Allergy Asthma Rep*. 2015; 15(9):53.

5. Olsson RF, Hagelberg S, Schiller B, Ringdén O, Truedsson L, Åhlin A. Allogeneic Hematopoietic Stem Cell Transplantation in the Treatment of Human C1q Deficiency: The Karolinska Experience. *Transplantation*. 2016; 100(6):1356–1362.

6. Schmidt RE, Grimbacher B, Witte T. Autoimmunity and primary immunodeficiency: two sides of the same coin?. *Nat Rev Rheumatol*. 2017; 14(1):7–18.

Family History and PID

PIDs are genetic diseases and most of them follow Mendelian pattern of inheritance (AD, AR, XL). A detailed family history is of paramount importance in arriving at an early diagnosis and guiding genetic evaluation in these patients.

Let me discuss few cases to highlight importance of family history.

Case 1

A 4-year-old boy was admitted with orbital cellulitis. Past history was non-contributory. Family history was significant. It was a non-consanguineous parentage. They had a 7-year-old healthy girl child, however, two male children had died at the age of 3 and 8. First child had recurrent ear discharge and died at the age of 3 due to meningitis. The second boy had repeated hospitalizations from the age of 2 and had succumbed to severe pneumonia at the age of 8.

The family history made us suspicious and we thought an X-linked disorder as only male children were affected in the family.

Investigations

✦ CBC: No neutropenia, lymphopenia or thrombocytopenia

Immunoglobulin profile was ordered:
✦ IgG <130 mg/dl
✦ IgA <30 mg/dl
✦ IgM <20 mg/dl

B cell counts: 0.5% (10–15%)

Genetic studies showed pathogenic mutation in the BTK gene.

Diagnosis: X-linked agammaglobulinemia

Case 2

A 5-month-old boy was admitted with history of fever and rapid breathing for 2 weeks. He was diagnosed to have pneumonia and started on intravenous antibiotics. He had significant failure to thrive (current weight: 3 kg, birth weight: 2.9 kg). He had been hospitalized previously at 3 months of age and been treated for pneumonia.

Family: Non-consanguineous wedlock. Two girl children (5Y and 2Y) were healthy. No death of siblings. But on further enquiry, three maternal uncles had died in early infancy (cause not known) (Fig. 13.1).

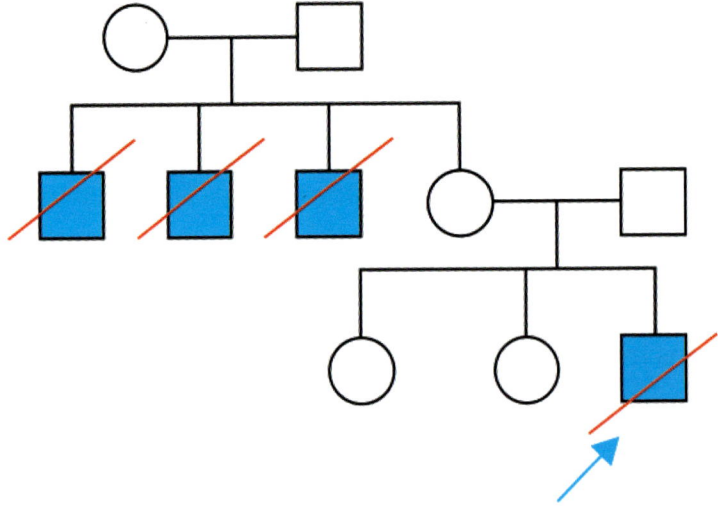

Fig. 13.1: Pedigree

Death of maternal uncles made us think of an X-linked pattern of inheritance.

Investigations

+ HIV rapid test: Negative
+ CBC: Hb—9 mg/dl, TC—13,000/mm^3 (N$_{84}$L$_6$ M$_6$ E$_4$), PC—123,000/mm^3
+ ANC: 10920, ALC: 780 (lymphopenia noted)

Immunological Work-up

+ IgG <130 mg/dl
+ IgA <17 mg/dl
+ IgM <15 mg/dl

Lymphocyte subsets: T—0.5%, B—95%, NK—1% (T-B+NK-)

Low immunoglobulins, absent T cells and X-linked pattern of inheritance/

Diagnosis: Severe combined immune deficiency (X-linked)

Genetic studies showed pathogenic mutation in IL2RG gene, confirming X-linked SCID.

Message
1. Early infantile deaths in family is a strong pointer towards a serious immune deficiency. One must always keep severe combined immune deficiency in mind in this context.
2. Think of X-linked pattern of inheritance if male siblings/maternal uncles/male maternal cousins are affected.

Case 3

An 8-year-old girl presented with fever and painful swelling in the right neck. Diagnosed with suppurative cervical lymphadenitis. Pus was drained and culture showed *Burkholderia cepacia*. She was treated with antibiotics based on the sensitivity.

Past history: She had been treated for liver abscess at the age of 3. She had undergone drainage of the liver abscess and had required a prolonged course of antibiotics.

Family history: Born to consanguineously married couple. Siblings (10-year-old boy, 5-year-old girl) were healthy.

In view of the unusual organism isolated during this admission, and the significant past history, she was evaluated further.

Investigations

+ HIV card test: Negative
+ CBC: Hb—9 g/dl, TC—24,500/mm^3 (N$_{75}$ L$_{15}$ M$_6$ E$_4$), PC—623,000/mm^3

+ ESR: 120 mm/1st hr
+ IgG: 2520 mg/dl (608–1572)
+ IgA: 230 mg/dl (33–236)
+ IgM: 324 mg/dl (43–207)
+ *Hypergammaglobulinemia noted.*
   NBT and DHR tests were performed and showed reduced oxidative burst.

Genetic studies: Homozygous pathogenic mutation in *NCF1* gene.

Diagnosis: Chronic granulomatous disease (AR inheritance).

Message:
1. Autosomal recessive diseases are more prevalent in families with consanguineous marriages.
2. 25% risk of recurrence in future pregnancies.

Case 4

A 14-year-old boy presented with fever for 3 weeks and severe backache. He was diagnosed to have vertebral osteomyelitis (involving L4 and L5 vertebra). Blood culture grew *Staphylococcus aureus*.

Past history: Hospitalized at the age of 3 for severe pneumonia and empyema. Repeated skin infections and eczema from the age of 5. Pathological fracture involving both bones of right forearm at the age of 10.

Family history: Non-consanguineous parentage. 3-year old sibling: Healthy.
   Father had been treated for severe pneumonia twice in the past; each episode required hospitalization for 7–10 days. He also had severe eczema from childhood and had coarse facies.

Investigations

+ CBC: Hb—10 g/dl, TC—14,300/mm^3 (N_{69} L_{15} $M_6 E_{10}$), PC—528,000/mm^3
+ AEC: 1430/mm^3
+ IgG—1220 mg/dl, IgA—156 mg/dl, IgM—130 mg/dl
+ IgE—3460 IU (<60)

Father was also evaluated.

+ IgG—1380 mg/dl, IgA—160 mg/dl, IgM—176 mg/dl
+ IgE—2345 IU (<60)

Autosomal dominant pattern of inheritance was suspected. With the clinical background and high IgE levels, hyper-IgE syndrome was considered. Genetic studies showed heterozygous mutation in STAT3 gene in the child and the father.

Diagnosis: AD hyper-IgE syndrome

Message

1. While children with very severe forms of immune deficiency (e.g. SCID) die in early childhood, others with milder immune defects survive into adulthood.
2. Autosomal dominant diseases have variable expressivity and thus two affected individuals within the same family may present with different degrees of severity of illness.

Did you know?

+ Survival of second child with SCID is better than the first child!
+ A family background of a child with SCID results in early diagnosis of SCID in the next child.

SUGGESTED READING

1. Chan A, Scalchunes C, Boyle M, Puck JM. Early vs. delayed diagnosis of severe combined immunodeficiency: a family perspective survey. *Clin Immunol.* 2011; 138(1):3–8. doi:10.1016/j.clim.2010.09.010

2. Hendaus MA, Alhammadi A, Adeli MM, Al-Yafei F. The value of family history in diagnosing primary immunodeficiency disorders. *Case Rep Pediatr.* 2014; 2014:516256.

3. Luk ADW, Lee PP, Mao H, et al. Family History of Early Infant Death Correlates with Earlier Age at Diagnosis But Not Shorter Time to Diagnosis for Severe Combined Immunodeficiency. *Front Immunol.* 2017; 8:808.

Lymphocyte Counts: An Important Clue to Serious Immune Deficiency

The complete hemogram is one of the most commonly requested investigations in clinical practice. Clinicians often give importance to total leukocyte counts (TC) and a high TC is most likely considered a sign of underlying infection. The presence of neutrophilia makes one think of sepsis and the entire focus is then directed to treat the presumed infection! We seldom make a note of lymphocyte counts, which may provide a very important clue for something sinister!

Let me share a true story.

A 4-month-old boy was hospitalized in a medical institute for the past 25 days. He had been running a high fever and had intermittent rashes. Past and family histories were unremarkable.

He was extensively evaluated for the cause of fever. Blood, urine and CSF cultures were sterile. HIV was excluded. Chest radiographs and ultrasound of the abdomen were reported normal. He failed to respond to the first line antibiotics, that were empirically upgraded to the second line. A bone marrow examination was carried out and reports came back normal.

We were completely lost and perplexed with what could be the diagnosis?

Residents are rotated between units (monthly at some medical institutes). A new resident took over the case the next month. He diligently went through all the records and made a diagnosis on the first day of his posting in the unit!!!

Eyes See Only What Mind Knows!

Let's have a look at the records.

CBC

Hb	9 g/dl	8.5	8.3	8.2
TC	9100/mm³	11000	10800	8900
PC	130,000/mm³	145,000	123,000	134,000

The new resident had a detailed look into the differential counts and here is what he found!

Hb	9	8.5	8.3	8.2
TC	9100	11000	10800	8900
DC	$N_{86}L_5M_5E_4$	$N_{80}L_8M_7E_5$	$N_{88}L_5M_5E_2$	$N_{78}L_9M_7E_6$
ANC	7826	8800	9504	6942
ALC	455	880	540	801
PC	130,000	145,000	123,000	134,000

Persistent lymphopenia across all the records!

He looked at the chest radiograph and the thymus was missing and he said "I have got the diagnosis. It is **severe combined immune deficiency!**".

Note: A relatively high lymphocyte percentage and counts is noted in healthy infants. With increasing age, neutrophilic predominance is anticipated.

Lymphopenia

Age	Absolute lymphocyte count
0–2 years	<3000/mm³
2–6 years	<1500/mm³
>6 years	<1000/mm³

Lymphocyte counts below 3000/mm³ in infancy must make one think of severe combined immune deficiency (SCID).

If lymphopenia is persistent, urgent evaluation is warranted as SCID is a medical emergency.

Message

1. Always look at the lymphocyte counts while evaluating sick infants.
2. Persistent lymphopenia is a strong pointer towards SCID in infants.
3. Children with SCID die in the first 2 years of life, unless they undergo a bone marrow transplant.

A Quick Look into the Disease

Severe combined immune deficiency

+ The most serious immune deficiency.
+ Characterized by absent T cells.
+ Presentation in early infancy and almost always within first year of life.
+ Clinical features: Pneumonia, diarrhea, ear discharge, oral thrush, failure to thrive.
+ (Note—if diagnosed early, these children would essentially look normal. With the onset of infections, they start failing to thrive)
+ Family history: History of sibling deaths in early infancy

Investigations

+ Lymphopenia (ALC <3000/mm³).
+ Low T cells and hypogammaglobulinemia.
+ Absent thymus (chest radiograph and ultrasound neck).
+ *Genetic testing:* More than a dozen genes have been implicated in SCID. Whole exome study by next generation sequencing must be carried out.
+ *Outcome:* 100% fatal in the absence of definitive treatment.
+ *Treatment:* Bone marrow transplant/hematopoietic stem cell transplant.

Did you know?

+ A lymphocyte keeps circulating through the blood and lymphatic system until it finds its specific antigen.

+ Each naïve T cell recirculates from blood through a lymph node and back to blood every 12 to 24 hours!

+ Lymphocytes multiply in peripheral tissues, neutrophils do not!

SUGGESTED READING

1. Aluri J, Desai M, Gupta M, et al. Clinical, Immunological, and Molecular Findings in 57 Patients with Severe Combined Immunodeficiency (SCID) From India. *Front Immunol*. 2019; 10:23.

2. Aluri J, Gupta MR, Dalvi A, et al. Lymphopenia and Severe Combined Immunodeficiency (SCID)—Think Before You Ink. *Indian J Pediatr*. 2019; 86(7):584–589.

3. Puck JM. Neonatal screening for severe combined immunodeficiency. *Curr Opin Pediatr*. 2011; 23(6):667–673.

4. Wekell P, Hertting O, Holmgren D, Fasth A. An overview of how on-call consultant paediatricians can recognise and manage severe primary immunodeficiencies. *Acta Paediatr*. 2019; 108(12):2175–2185.

Neutrophil Counts: Too Less and Too Many— Both can be Immune Deficiency!

Conventionally, neutrophilic leukocytosis in a child with fever is attributed to an infection (most likely a bacterial infection). However, presence of low neutrophil counts is unusual and must be given due attention.

Neutropenia

>1 year	ANC <1500/mm^3
<1 year	ANC <2000/mm^3

Classification of Congenital Neutropenia

Classification	*ANC*
Mild neutropenia	1000–1500/mm^3
Moderate neutropenia	500–1000/mm^3
Severe neutropenia	<500/mm^3
Persistent neutropenia	ANC always <1500/mm^3
Intermittent neutropenia	ANC occasionally <1500/mm^3
Cyclic neutropenia	ANC with periodic oscillations and nadir <1000/mm^3

Children presenting with persistent or recurrent neutropenia must be evaluated for underlying PID.

Let me explain with few clinical cases.

Case 1

A 4-month-old girl child, product of second degree consanguinity, presented with draining ears from second month of life. She was now hospitalized with severe pneumonia.

Family history: First born. No history of sibling deaths.

Investigations

+ CBC: Hb—8.5 g/dl, TC—7,300/mm^3 (**N$_9$** L$_{80}$ M$_6$ E$_5$), PC—523,000/mm^3
+ ANC: 657/mm^3

Previous records were reviewed
+ CBC: Hb—9 g/dl, TC—5,200/mm^3 (N$_5$ L$_{75}$ M$_{15}$ E$_5$), PC—236,000/mm^3
+ ANC: 260/mm^3
+ CBC: Hb—9.2 g/dl, TC—6,500/mm^3 (N$_7$ L$_{78}$ M$_{12}$ E$_3$), PC—639,000/mm^3
+ ANC: 455/mm^3

Neutrophils were persistently reduced. Intermittent monocytosis was noted. Hematologist was consulted and a decision to perform bone marrow examination was taken.

Bone marrow biopsy: Maturation arrest in the myeloid lineage (only precursors in the myeloid lineage were seen). Erythroid and megakaryocytic lineages were normal.

Diagnosis: Severe congenital neutropenia

Genetic studies: Pathogenic mutation in ELANE gene.

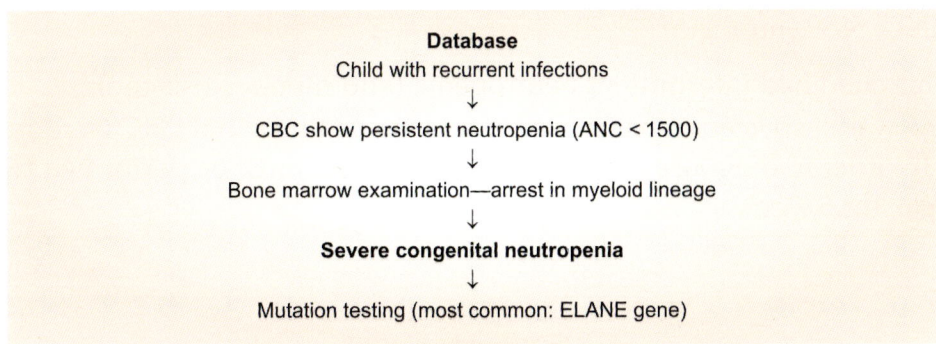

Database
Child with recurrent infections
↓
CBC show persistent neutropenia (ANC < 1500)
↓
Bone marrow examination—arrest in myeloid lineage
↓
Severe congenital neutropenia
↓
Mutation testing (most common: ELANE gene)

A Quick Look into the Disease

Severe congenital neutropenia
+ Heterogenous group of disorders characterized by persistent neutropenia
+ ANC <1500 (and mostly below 500)
+ Severe infections in early childhood (pneumonia, otitis media, mastoiditis)
+ Bone marrow examination: Arrest in myeloid lineage
+ Mutations in ELANE, HAX1, WAS, SBDS, SLC37A4, G6PC3, etc.
+ *Treatment:* G-CSF therapy, bone marrow transplant

Case 2

A 7-year-old girl presented with recurrent episodes of oral ulcers. These ulcers would last for 3–5 days and recur almost monthly. She had been hospitalized twice for pneumonia. Also had had ear discharge last year.

She had undergone multiple blood tests and when the records were analysed, the following was noted.

+ CBC: Hb—10.2 g/dl, TC—5,200/mm³ (N_5 L_{75} M_{15} E_5), PC—436,000/mm³
+ ANC: 260/mm³

+ CBC: Hb—10 g/dl, TC—8,200/mm³ (N_{65} L_{25} M_{05} E_5), PC—239,000/mm³
+ ANC: 5330/mm³

+ CBC: Hb—9.2 g/dl, TC—6,500/mm³ (N_7 L_{78} M_{12} E_3), PC—539,000/mm³
+ ANC: 455/mm³

+ CBC: Hb—9 g/dl, TC—7,500/mm³ (N_{78} L_{12} M_7 E_3), PC—639,000/mm³
+ ANC: 5850/mm³

This child had intermittent neutropenia (and monocytosis too).

She was suspected to have cyclic neutropenia and serial CBC were asked for. In order to diagnose cyclic neutropenia, CBC must be performed twice a week for 6 weeks.

Date	Hb (g/dl)	TC (per mm³)	DC	PC (per mm³)	ANC (per mm³)
1st June	10	7600	$N_{60}L_{30}M_6E_4$	450,000	4560
4th June	10.2	6500	$N_{45}L_{40}M_8E_7$	300,000	2925
7th June	9.5	4000	$N_5L_{65}M_{25}E_5$	230,000	200
10th June	9.8	4200	$N_{10}L_{60}M_{20}E_7B_3$	200,000	420
13th June	10	6700	$N_{45}L_{50}M_3E_2$	223,000	3015
16th June	10.3	7000	$N_{67}L_{25}M_6E_2$	350,000	4690
19th June	10.5	8700	$N_{70}L_{22}M_5E_3$	340,000	6090
22nd June	10	7700	$N_{58}L_{25}M_9E_6B_2$	245,000	4466
25th June	10.2	8340	$N_{35}L_{55}M_5E_5$	234,000	2905
28th June	9.4	4100	$N_3L_{60}M_{27}E_7B_3$	165,000	123
1st July	10.3	4500	$N_{10}L_{62}M_{20}E_6B_2$	187,000	450
4th July	10.2	8000	$N_{68}L_{24}M_6E_2$	289,000	5440

Note: ANC dropped to less than 1000 mm³ on two occasions (3 weeks apart).

Diagnosis: Cyclic neutropenia

Genetic testing: Pathogenic mutation in ELANE gene

A Quick Look into the Disease

Cyclic neutropenia
+ Neutropenia occurs once in 21–25 days.
+ Neutropenia lasts for 3–5 days.
+ During periods of neutropenia, children develop oral mucositis, infections (otitis media, pneumonia, etc.).

+ Bone marrow examination just before the expected time of neutropenia: Arrest in myeloid lineage.
+ Mutations in ELANE gene.
+ *Treatment:* G-CSF therapy.

Do Very High Neutrophil Counts Point towards a PID?

Have you seen children with total white cell counts of >1,00,000/mm³?

I am sure you would have thought of leukemia or a leukamoid reaction in these cases. But most often these children would have a marked lymphocytosis and the diagnosis in those cases would be acute lymphoblastic leukemia.

But have you seen a child with WBC counts >1,00,000/mm³ and neutrophilic predominance?

Let me discuss a case.

A 9-month-old girl presented with chronic diarrhea for the past 3 months. She had developed perianal ulcers. She had been hospitalized at multiple places and investigated. As she had persistent leukocytosis, she was thought to have sepsis and given variety of antibiotics, but with no relief.

She was referred to our department with a suspicion of PID. Her previous records were analyzed.

+ CBC: Hb—10.2 g/dl, TC—92,000/mm³ (N_{85} L_{10} M_4 E_1), PC—536,000/mm³
+ ANC: 78,200/mm³

+ CBC: Hb—10 g/dl, TC—108,200/mm³ (N_{82} L_{12} M_5 E_1), PC—139,000/mm³
+ ANC: 88,560/mm³

+ CBC: Hb—9.2 g/dl, TC—86,500/mm³ (N_{87} L_8 M_3 E_2), PC—465,000/mm³
+ ANC: 75,255/mm³

+ CBC: Hb—9 g/dl, TC—67,500/mm³ (N_{82} L_{10} M_7 E_1), PC—639,000/mm³
+ ANC: 55,350/mm³

This child had persistent neutrophilic leukocytosis and the counts remained high even when the child was clinically well. Is this the pattern that you note in sepsis? The answer is NO.

Persistent severe neutrophilia in a child with recurrent infections—think of leukocyte adhesion deficiency (LAD)

Further Investigations

✦ CD18 expression on neutrophils was studied by flow cytometry.
✦ CD18 0.1 % (normal—99%)

Diagnosis: Leukocyte adhesion deficiency type 1

Database
Child with recurrent infections/non-healing ulcers
↓
CBC show persistently high neutrophil counts (ANC > 20,000)
↓
Leukocyte adhesion deficiency
↓
CD18 expression reduced on neutrophils (flow cytometry)

A Quick Look into the Disease

Leukocyte adhesion deficiency
✦ Group of genetic disorders characterized by defect in adhesion of neutrophils to the endothelium of blood vessels
✦ Autosomal recessive inheritance
✦ Clinical features: Delay in fall of umbilical cord, omphalitis, perianal ulcers, recurrent pneumonia, diarrhea
✦ No pus formation
✦ *CBC:* Very high neutrophil counts
   White cell counts may be as high as 1,00,000/mm^3.
✦ *LAD I:* Absent CD18 expression on neutrophils, mutation in *ITGB2* gene.
✦ *LAD II:* Absent CD15a expression on neutrophils, Bombay blood group, mutation in GDP- fucose transporter gene
✦ *LAD III:* Defect in integrin activation, mutation in *FERMT3* gene

Did you know?

The normal neutrophil count is about 3 to 7.5 billion per liter of blood, but having at least 1.5 billion per liter usually provides an adequate defence against life-threatening infection. Due to their short lifespan, the bone marrow must produce about one hundred billion neutrophils per day to have enough neutrophils in the blood and tissues. That means the body makes about one million neutrophils per second!

SUGGESTED READING

1. Almarza Novoa E, Kasbekar S, Thrasher AJ, et al. Leukocyte adhesion deficiency-I: A comprehensive review of all published cases. *J Allergy Clin Immunol Pract*. 2018; 6(4):1418–1420.

2. Dale DC, Bolyard AA, Aprikyan A. Cyclic neutropenia. *Semin Hematol*. 2002; 39(2):89–94.

3. Dale DC, Welte K. Cyclic and chronic neutropenia. *Cancer Treat Res*. 2011; 157:97–108.

4. Etzioni A. Leukocyte adhesion deficiency III—when integrins activation fails. *J Clin Immunol*. 2014; 34(8):900–903.

5. Justiz Vaillant AA, Ahmad F. Leukocyte Adhesion Deficiency. In: *StatPearls*. Treasure Island (FL): StatPearls Publishing; 2020.

6. Spoor J, Farajifard H, Rezaei N. Congenital neutropenia and primary immunodeficiency diseases. *Crit Rev Oncol Hematol*. 2019; 133:149–162.

Immunoglobulin Assay and Clinical Correlation

Immunoglobulins/antibodies are proteins produced by B cells and play a pivotal role in the defense of the body against infections. Activated B cells (plasma cells) secrete one of the four major classes of antibody: IgM, IgA, IgG, and IgE. Immunoglobulin IgD is only secreted in small amounts and its function remains unclear. Hence in clinical practice, we often ask for IgG, IgA, IgM, and IgE levels.

IgG antibodies are the most common isotype in the serum. They include four subclasses—IgG1, IgG2, IgG3, and IgG4. IgG2 is important in handling encapsulated bacteria (e.g. *Pneumococcus*).

Children and adults with a deficiency of immunoglobulin production are at risk of recurrent infections. These groups of disorders are called humoral immune deficiencies.

Let us discuss a few cases.

Case 1

A 4-year-old boy was referred with a history of recurrent chest infections. He had had 4 episodes of pneumonia, requiring admission and IV antibiotics (first episode at the age of 8 months). He also had 2 episodes of ear discharge.

He had been previously evaluated for recurrent pneumonia.

Common differentials considered while evaluating children with recurrent pneumonia are:
1. Congenital heart disease (left to right shunts)
2. Congenital lung anomaly (e.g. congenital lobar emphysema)

3. Aspiration syndromes (e.g. gastroesophageal reflux disease)
4. Ciliary dyskinesia
5. Cystic fibrosis

The index case had been extensively evaluated elsewhere before he was referred to our department.

+ Echocardiography: Normal
+ CT chest: Normal
+ Sweat chloride study: Normal
+ GER scan: No reflux

Family history: Non-contributory

Examination

Throat examination: Tonsils were absent!

Further evaluation:
Immunoglobulins were performed.
+ IgG <130 mg/dl
+ IgA <20 mg/dl
+ IgM <30 mg/dl

B cell counts: 1% (10–15%)

Genetic testing: Mutation in BTK gene

Diagnosis: X-linked agammaglobulinemia

Case 2

A 36-year-old gentleman referred by the pulmonologist to immunology services. He had been admitted thrice in the previous year and had received treatment for pneumonia during each of this admissions.

Past history: recurrent sinusitis from the age of 10.

We performed serum immunoglobulins.
+ IgG: 270 mg/dl (639–1349)
+ IgA: <26 mg/dl (70–312)
+ IgM: 35 mg/dl (56–352)

Lymphocyte Subsets
+ CD3: 71% (50–75)

+ CD19: 15% (10–15)

+ CD56: 12% (5–10)

Diagnosis: Common variable immune deficiency

Case 3

A 3-year-old boy presented with the 3rd episode of severe pneumonia. He had been ventilated for 10 days during the first episode at the age of 6 months. After extensive evaluation (echocardiography, CT chest, Cystic fibrosis work up), he was referred to immunology department.

We looked at the immunoglobulin profile

+ IgG: <27 mg/dl

+ IgA: <20 mg/dl

+ **IgM:>530 mg/dl**

B cell counts: Normal

Diagnosis: Hyper-IgM syndrome

Genetic testing: Mutation in CD40L gene, confirming hyper-IgM syndrome type 1.

From the above three cases, it must clear that immunoglobulin assay is mandatory in children and adults presenting with recurrent infections. Often, these patients are subjected to a battery of investigations (non-invasive and invasive) and do not find a solution to the ongoing issues. An immunoglobulin profile that is readily available to most physicians can be of diagnostic value.

Caution: Always look at the age norms while interpreting immunoglobulin reports. Most labs provide normative data only for adults and this is irrelevant to the pediatric population.

Message

Immunological profile	Likely diagnosis	Comments
Low IgG, IgA and IgM and absent B cells in a boy	X-linked agammaglobulinemia	Absent tonsils is a clinical clue.
Low IgG, IgA and/or IgM and normal B cells	Common variable immune deficiency (CVID)	This is a diagnosis of exclusion and other causes of low immunoglobulins must be considered before making a diagnosis of CVID.
Low IgG, IgA and high IgM	Hyper-IgM syndrome	50% of children with hyper-IgM syndrome have normal IgM levels; hence low IgG, IgA and normal IgM could be consistent with hyper-IgM syndrome.
High IgG	Hypergammaglobulinemia	Seen in HIV infection, autoimmune and inflammatory diseases. Chronic granulomatous disease often presents with high IgG levels.
High IgE levels	Immune deficiencies that can present with high IgE—hyper-IgE syndrome (AD), due to STAT3 mutation; Hyper-IgE syndrome (AR), due to DOCK8 mutation; Wiskott-Aldrich syndrome; Omenn syndrome.	
IgG is low, while other immunoglobulins are normal. B cell counts are normal.	Transient hypogamma-globulinemia of infancy.	Response to vaccines (anti-diphtheria titres are normal). Most of them resolve by the age of 4.

Did you know?

+ Immunoglobulin assay costs less than a CT chest! Think about it, before you expose a child to the radiation!

+ IgM is normal (not high) in 50% of cases with hyper-IgM syndrome.

SUGGESTED READING

1. Abolhassani H, Sagvand BT, Shokuhfar T, Mirminachi B, Rezaei N, Aghamohammadi A. A review on guidelines for management and treatment of common variable immunodeficiency. *Expert Rev Clin Immunol.* 2013; 9(6):561–575.

2. Agarwal S, Cunningham-Rundles C. Assessment and clinical interpretation of reduced IgG values. *Ann Allergy Asthma Immunol.* 2007; 99(3):281–283.

3. El-Sayed ZA, Abramova I, Aldave JC, et al. X-linked agammaglobulinemia (XLA):Phenotype, diagnosis, and therapeutic challenges around the world. *World Allergy Organ J.* 2019; 12(3):100018.

4. Tam JS, Routes JM. Common variable immunodeficiency. *Am J Rhinol Allergy.* 2013; 27(4):260–265.

IgG Subclass Deficiency

A 10-year-old girl presented with recurrent rhino-sinusitis and repeated episodes of pneumonia. She had been hospitalized on at least three occasions so far. Blood culture grew *Streptococcus pneumoniae* on one occassion. Extensive evaluation for the cause of repeated infections (including CT chest, echocardiography etc) was non-rewarding.

We suspected a humoral immune defect and performed an immuno-globulin profile:

+ IgG: 1650 mg/dl (608–1572)
+ IgA: 10 mg/dl (33–236)
+ IgM: 110 mg/dl (52–242)
+ IgA was reduced and IgG was high!

So, the diagnosis considered was IgA deficiency.

However, IgA deficiency is known to present with a milder phenotype (repeated rhinitis, sinusitis). This child had recurrent pneumonia and hence further evaluation was considered.

IgG subclass estimation was ordered.

+ IgG1: 1425 mg/dl (423–939)
+ **IgG2: 45 mg/dl (70–426)**
+ IgG3: 150 mg/dl (27–207)
+ IgG4: 27 mg/dl (8–32)

Diagnosis: IgG2 subclass deficiency with IgA deficiency

Note: IgA should be less than 14 mg/dl to qualify for a partial IgA deficiency and less than 7 mg/dl to qualify for complete IgA deficiency in a child 4 or older.

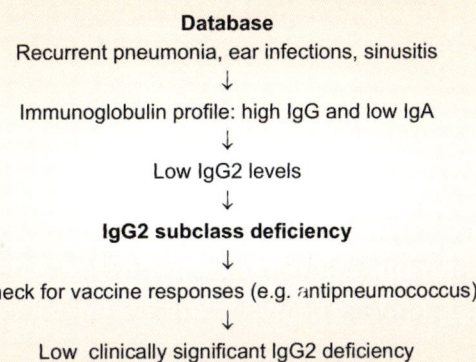

Database
Recurrent pneumonia, ear infections, sinusitis
↓
Immunoglobulin profile: high IgG and low IgA
↓
Low IgG2 levels
↓
IgG2 subclass deficiency
↓
Check for vaccine responses (e.g. antipneumococcus)
↓
Low clinically significant IgG2 deficiency

A Quick Look into the Disease

IgG2 subclass deficiency

+ IgG2 is essential in immune response against encapsulated bacteria.
+ IgG2 deficiency presents with recurrent upper and lower respiratory tract infections with *Pneumococcus, H. influenzae* and other encapsulated bacteria.
+ Children with IgG2 deficiency can be IgA deficient.
+ Functional assessment (post-vaccination antibody titres) is necessary to define clinically significant deficiency.
+ Treatment
   a. Antibiotic prophylaxis (co-trimoxazole)
   b. Vaccination with conjugate pneumoccal vaccine followed by polysaccharide vaccine
   c. If the child continues to have recurrent infections despite above measures, immunoglobulin infusion (IVIG).

Message

1. Recurrent upper and lower respiratory tract infections—Normal Immunoglobulin profile—look for IgG2 deficiency
2. Severe infections in a child with low IgA—look for IgG2 deficiency
3. Long term follow-up is essential, as children with IgA deficiency and IgG2 deficiency can evolve into common variable immune deficiency (CVID).

Did you know?

Excess of IgG4 is associated with a group of diseases called "IgG4-related disorders." A group of fibro-inflammatory diseases, usually responsive to steroids, e.g. pseudotumors of liver, kidney, GIT, recurrent pancreatitis, etc.

SUGGESTED READING

1. Kim JH, Park S, Hwang YI, et al. Immunoglobulin G Subclass Deficiencies in Adult Patients with Chronic Airway Diseases. *J Korean Med Sci.* 2016; 31(10):1560–1565. doi:10.3346/jkms.2016.31.10.1560.

2. Nettagul R, Visitsunthorn N, Vichyanond P. A case of IgG subclass deficiency with the initial presentation of transient hypogammaglobulinemia of infancy and a review of IgG subclass deficiencies. *J Med Assoc Thai.* 2003; 86(7):686–692.

3. Parker AR, Skold M, Ramsden DB, Ocejo-Vinyals JG, López-Hoyos M, Harding S. The Clinical Utility of Measuring IgG Subclass Immunoglobulins During Immunological Investigation for Suspected Primary Antibody Deficiencies. *Lab Med.* 2017; 48(4):314–325. doi:10.1093/labmed/lmx058.

4. Rawat A, Suri D, Gupta A, Saikia B, Minz RW, Singh S. Isolated immunoglobulin G4 subclass deficiency in a child with bronchiectasis. *Indian J Pediatr.* 2014; 81(9):932–933.

Lymphocyte Subsets

Immunological testing often involves enumeration of T cell, B cell and NK cell counts. Let us understand them in more detail.

Cells can be recognized by surface proteins they express and this is the principle of flow cytometry (kindly refer standard textbooks to understand in depth about flow cytometry).

Markers for different lymphocytes are as follows:

+ T cells—CD3
+ B cells—CD19
+ NK cells—CD56

Note:

T cells also express several other markers (CD4, CD8, etc.).

B cells also express CD20.

NK cells also express CD16.

Helper and Cytotoxic T Cells

There are two major types of T cells in the body:

+ Helper T cells : CD3+ CD4+
+ Cytotoxic T cells : CD3+ CD8+

While B cells produce antibodies, T cell help is very crucial for normal B cell function. Hence if T cells are absent, immunoglobulins would be reduced, despite a good B cell number.

Example: Severe combined immune deficiency (SCID)

In one of the subtypes of SCID, T and NK cells are absent, while B cells are present (T-B+NK-) and these children have hypogammaglobulinemia.

It is also essential to understand that B cells produce IgM in response to an infection, but at a later point, these B cells switch to produce IgG, IgA, and IgE. This is called class switching. Interaction between T cells and B cells is necessary to produce class switching (CD40L on T cells interact with CD40 on B cells). If CD40L or CD40 is deficient, B cells keep producing only IgM. This is called hyper-IgM syndrome.

When do you look at the lymphocyte subsets?

Case 1

A 3-year-old boy presented with recurrent episodes of pneumonia and discharging ears. On evaluation, immunoglobulins (IgG, IgA and IgM) were markedly reduced.

In this setting, one would be interested to look at the B cell counts.

Further, lymphocyte subsets showed low B cells.
Absolute lymphocyte counts—3500/mm³

CD3–85% (50–70%)	CD3 counts—2975/mm³ (1222–3790)
CD19–0.2% (10–15%)	CD19 counts—7/mm³ (88–1576)
CD56–13% (5–10%)	CD56 counts—455/mm³ (54–261)

The most likely diagnosis in this child is X-linked agammaglobulinemia.

Case 2

A 4-month-old girl presented with persistent oral thrush and failure to thrive. She had an episode of pneumonia and was hospitalized.

Few salient features in this case:
a. Onset of illness in early infancy (<6 months of age)
b. Oral candidiasis
c. Failure to thrive

These features point towards a T cell defect.

Lymphocyte subsets

+ CD3: 2 % (50–70%)
+ CD19: 91% (10–15%)
+ CD56: 3 % (5–10%)

Markedly reduced T cells in this setting confirm a diagnosis of severe combined immune deficiency (SCID).

Severe Combined Immune Deficiency (SCID)

T cells are reduced in number while B and NK cells may be normal or reduced.

By definition,
T cell < 20% (absolute CD3 < –2SD for age)

Note: CD3 < 300/mm^3 is diagnostic.

The immunological phenotype may give a clue regarding the underlying genetic defect:

Table 18.1:	
Lymphocyte subsets	**Type of SCID**
T- B- NK-	ADA deficiency
T- B+ NK-	IL2RG, JAK3
T- B- NK+	RAG1, RAG2, DCLRE1C, DNA Ligase IV, Cernunnos
T- B+ NK+	IL7Rα, Coronin 1a

(Variants of SCID with normal T cell counts—Omenn syndrome, maternal T cell engraftment)

CD4 and CD8 counts

Low CD4 counts can be seen in

+ HIV infection
+ MHC class II deficiency
+ Idiopathic CD4 lymphocytopenia

Low CD8 counts can be seen in ZAP70 deficiency.

Note: Always look at the absolute counts (and not only %) while analysing lymphocyte subsets.

Did you know?

+ NKT cells are innate-like T lymphocytes that recognize glycolipid antigens presented by the MHC class I-like protein CD1d.
+ These cells share surface markers and functional characteristics with both conventional T lymphocytes and natural killer cells.
+ Low NKT cells have been noted in patients with XLP (X-linked lymphoproliferative disease).

SUGGESTED READING

1. Amatuni GS, Sciortino S, Currier RJ, Naides SJ, Church JA, Puck JM. Reference intervals for lymphocyte subsets in preterm and term neonates without immune defects. *J Allergy Clin Immunol*. 2019; 144(6):1674–1683.

2. Madkaikar MR, Shabrish S, Kulkarni M, et al. Application of Flow Cytometry in Primary Immunodeficiencies: Experience from India. *Front Immunol*. 2019; 10:1248.

3. Pasquier B, Yin L, Fondanèche MC, et al. Defective NKT cell development in mice and humans lacking the adapter SAP, the X-linked lymphoproliferative syndrome gene product. *J Exp Med*. 2005; 201(5):695–701.

4. Rawat A, Arora K, Shandilya J, et al. Flow Cytometry for Diagnosis of Primary Immune Deficiencies-A Tertiary Center Experience From North India. *Front Immunol*. 2019; 10:2111.

NBT and DHR Tests

Phagocytosis and Intracellular Killing

Neutrophils play an important role in handling infections (bacterial and fungal). Following phagocytosis of organisms, intracellular killing is carried out by free radicals (reactive oxygen species) generated by the NADPH oxidase complex. This process is called the oxidative burst and a defect in NADPH oxidase hampers this process, resulting in an increased risk of bacterial and fungal infections. Defect in NADPH oxidase causes chronic granulomatous disease (CGD). Nitroblue tetrazolium test (NBT) and dihydrorhodamine test (DHR) are screening tests for CGD.

Nitroblue Tetrazolium Test (NBT)

Principle

NBT is a yellow dye and when reduced (oxido-reduction reaction), produces blue–black formazan granules. In NBT test, neutrophils are stimulated (using yeast/PMA) and tested for production of formazan granules.

Types

1. Yeast—stimulated NBT
2. PMA—stimulated NBT (PMA, phorbol myristate acetate)

Procedure

Yeast—stimulated NBT

Materials needed

1. Heparinized blood
2. NBT dye
3. Yeast powder
4. Slides
5. Microscope
6. Incubator

Preparation

+ Yeast solution is prepared 2 hours prior to the actual test. 5 ml of yeast solution is prepared in a strength of 2 mg/ml. Vortex intermittently.
+ NBT dye solution is prepared only prior to the test, in a strength of 1 mg/ml (in normal saline).
+ Two slides are labeled as US—unstimulated and S—stimulated.

The Test

+ 2 ml of fresh heparinized blood is taken and allowed to settle at room temperature. As the supernatant becomes clear (free of RBCs), 30 η|F of supernatant is taken and added over the slides (30 η|F over the US slide and 30 η|F over the S slide)
+ 30 μl of NBT solution is added to both the slides.
+ 30 μl of yeast solution is added only to the S slide.

The slides are incubated in a moist chamber at 37°C for 30 minutes. Thereafter, the slides are studied under microscope.

Results

100 neutrophils are counted in each slide (US and S). The US slide appears yellow. In case of healthy sample, the S slide would show engulfment of yeast cells by neutrophils and formation of blue–black pigment in most of the neutrophils (Fig. 19.1).

In case of CGD sample, the S slide does not form (or very minimal) blue–black pigment. The yeast cells however would be engulfed by the neutrophils.

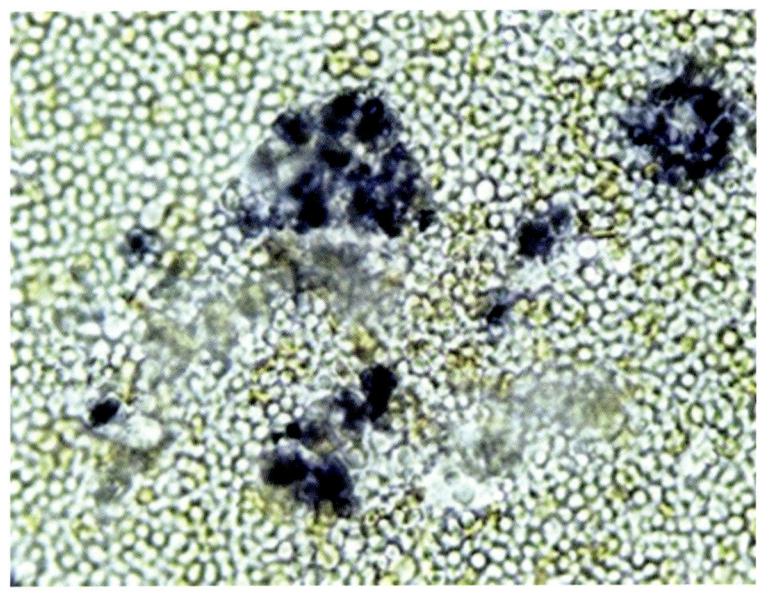

Fig. 19.1: Bluish–black pigment (formazan granules) formation in S slide indicates normal oxidative burst.

NBT test is thus a very simple and cost-effective test for diagnosis of CGD, however, it is observer-dependent. DHR test is more objective and is the screening test of choice where facilities for flow cytometry are available.

Sample copy of the NBT result would be as follows:

Report/C/A		What does it mean?
Control	**Unstimulated—5%**	5% neutrophils show pigment
Control	**Stimulated—90%**	90% neutrophils show pigment
Patient	**Unstimulated—0 %**	No cells show pigment
Patient	**Stimulated—0%**	No cells show pigment

Dihydrorhodamine (DHR) Test

Principle

+ Flow cytometry based test.
+ Neutrophils are stimulated (PMA is the stimulant) and DHR is oxidized to produce rhodamine, which is fluorescent. The degree of fluorescence defines the function of the neutrophils.

Procedure

3 tubes (Fig. 19.2)
   1. Heparinized blood
   2. Heparinized blood + DHR
   3. Heparinized blood + DHR + PMA

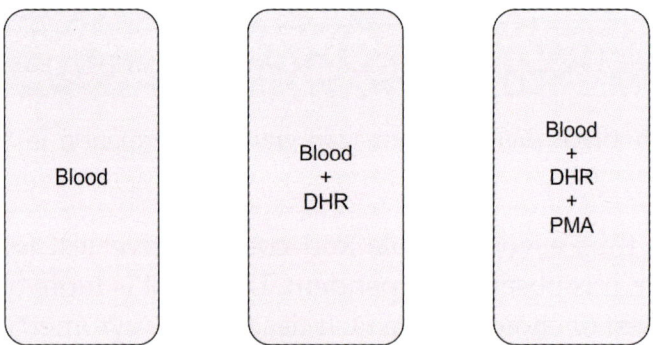

Fig. 19.2: Three tubes with blood, blood with DHR and blood with DHR and PMA respectively

Neutrophils are stimulated with PMA (phorbol myristate acetate). In a healthy sample, superoxide anion produced due to respiratory burst would oxidize dihydrorhodamine (DHR) to rhodamine, which is fluorescent. This increase in fluorescence is calculated in the form of stimulation index (SI) or oxidative index (OI).

   SI = MFI of stimuated sample/MFI of unstimulated sample
   (MFI—median fluorescence intensity)

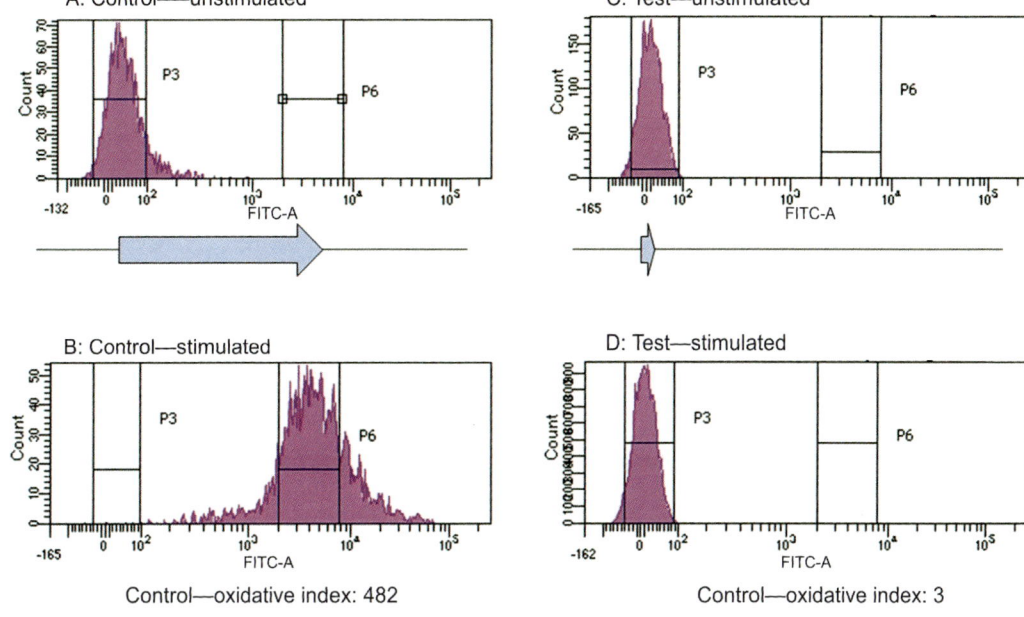

Fig. 19.3

Panel A and B = Control (unstimulated and stimulated)
                  Oxidative index 482
Panel C and D = Test (unstimulated and stimulated)
                  Oxidative index 3
An oxidative index <30 is considered to be abnormal.
{Control—sample from a healthy person, test—sample from a child with CGD}

Did you know?

Elie Metchnikoff discovered phagocytes and was awarded Noble Prize for his contribution to the science of immunity.

SUGGESTED READING

1. El-Benna J, Hurtado-Nedelec M, Marzaioli V, Marie JC, Gougerot-Pocidalo MA, Dang PM. Priming of the neutrophil respiratory burst: Role in host defense and inflammation. *Immunol Rev.* 2016; 273(1):180–193.

2. Jirapongsananuruk O, Malech HL, Kuhns DB, et al. Diagnostic paradigm for evaluation of male patients with chronic granulomatous disease, based on the dihydrorhodamine 123 assay. *J Allergy Clin Immunol.* 2003; 111(2):374–379.

3. Kulkarni M, Gupta M, Madkaikar M. Phenotypic Prenatal Diagnosis of Chronic Granulomatous Disease: A Useful Tool in The Absence of Molecular Diagnosis. *Scand J Immunol.* 2017; 86(6):486–490.

4. Rawat A, Bhattad S, Singh S. Chronic Granulomatous Disease. *Indian J Pediatr.* 2016; 83(4):345–353.

Naïve T cells and Recent Thymic Emigrants

> **Have your T cells got educated?**
> **Have they been to the University of Thymus?**

T cells produced from the bone marrow undergo extensive training in thymus. During this process, auto-reactive T cells are deleted. T cells that are released from the thymus are called the **recent thymic emigrants (RTE).** They represent the thymic output.

With advancing age, there is a physiological reduction in the thymic output and hence proportion of RTE get reduced as well.

T cells that have not encountered antigens are called the **naïve T cells.** Newborns would have high percentage of naïve T cells.

Markers

✦ Naïve helper T cells—CD3/CD4/CD62L/CD45RA
✦ RTE—CD4/CD31/CD45RA

Clinical Application

In a child suspected to have SCID, CD3 <300/mm^3 is diagnostic of SCID (CD3 <20% of the total lymphocytes). This has been discussed in depth in Chapter 18.

Occasionally, CD3 counts are low (< –2 SD for age), however they are above 300/mm^3 (or > 20% of the total lymphocytes). In such cases, diagnosis of SCID becomes challenging. One can perform T-cell proliferation assay in this setting. Absence of T-cell proliferation would confirm SCID, however, these tests are not readily available.

In all such cases, where the results seem borderline, we must assess the thymic output. A low thymic output (reduced RTE and/or low naïve T cells) would be suggestive of SCID.

Let me explain with a case.

A 9-month-old boy presented with chronic diarrhea for past 3 months, recurrent oral thrush and failure to thrive.

Evaluation

+ HIV card test—non-reactive
+ CBC showed lymphopenia (ALC 2000/mm³)

Immunoglobulins

+ IgG: 220 mg/dl (172–1069)
+ IgA <20 (11–106)
+ IgM <30 (33–126)
+ CD3: 32%, CD3 counts—640 cells/mm³ (1900–5900)
+ CD19: 5%, CD19 counts—100 cells/mm³ (610–2600)
+ CD56: 63%, CD56 counts—1260 cells/mm³ (160–950)

In this particular case, SCID is high on cards. T cells are low in number but >300/mm³. It is very essential to confirm the diagnosis, before the child is taken up for a bone marrow transplant.

Naïve T cells and RTE were asked for.

Naïve Helper T Cells

CD3 + CD4 + CD62L + CD45 RA + = 12% (normal—58–91% at 9 months of age)

Recent Thymic Emigrants

CD4 + CD31 + CD45 RA = 5% of CD4 + T cells (normal—65–90 % at 9 months of age).

Both naïve T cells and RTE were markedly reduced, indicating poor thymic output.

Later, genetic studies confirmed mutation in RAG1 gene.

Final diagnosis: SCID due to RAG1 deficiency.

Message
1. Assessment of thymic output (naïve T cell counts and/or recent thymic emigrants) would be useful in cases suspected of having SCID (with presence of few T cells).
2. In children with SCID, immune reconstitution following a BMT can be assessed by monitoring recent thymic emigrants.

Did you know?
95% of thymocytes die during their transit in thymus!
"A difficult journey indeed".

SUGGESTED READING

1. Cunningham CA, Helm EY, Fink PJ. Reinterpreting recent thymic emigrant function: defective or adaptive? *Curr Opin Immunol*. 2018; 51:1–6.

2. Kurd N, Robey EA. T-cell selection in the thymus: a spatial and temporal perspective. *Immunol Rev*. 2016; 271(1):114–126.

3. Seo W, Taniuchi I. Transcriptional regulation of early T-cell development in the thymus. *Eur J Immunol*. 2016; 46(3):531–538.

4. Sprent J, Surh CD. Normal T cell homeostasis: the conversion of naive cells into memory-phenotype cells. *Nat Immunol*. 2011; 12(6):478–484.

Genetic Tests to Diagnose Immune Deficiency

The majority of the PIDs are monogenic disorders and follow a Mendelian pattern of inheritance. Clinical history and a detailed family history is thereby very crucial to understand the kind of inheritance one is looking at in a given case.

+ Consanguinity in parents—likely autosomal recessive disease.
+ Male siblings/maternal uncles being affected—likely X-linked recessive disease.
+ If one of the parents is also affected—likely autosomal dominant disease.

Various platforms for genetic testing are:
1. Karyotyping
2. Fluorescent *in-situ* hybridization (FISH)
3. Comparative genomic hybridization (CGH)
4. Sanger sequencing
5. Next generation sequencing (NGS)

A detailed discussion on various genetic testing platforms is beyond the scope of this book and interested readers can refer to standard textbooks on genetics. I would attempt to highlight the facts a clinician must know before ordering a genetic test.

Why Perform a Genetic Test?

1. To confirm the diagnosis at the molecular level.
2. To provide targeted therapy.

3. To predict risk of recurrence in the next pregnancy and offer antenatal testing.

For simplicity, genetic diseases can be broadly classified into:
a. Chromosomal disorders and
b. Mendelian disorders.

Chromosomal disorders: Abnormal number or structure of chromosomes. For example, down syndrome (trisomy 21). Karyotyping, FISH and CGH are useful in the diagnosis of chromosomal disorders.

Mendelian disorders: Single gene diseases. Sanger sequencing and NGS are useful in the diagnosis of Mendelian disorders.

> **Note:** Majority of PIDs are Mendelian disorders.

Let us have a look at the various genetic testing platforms and understand them with few clinical examples:

1. **Karyotyping:** Microscopic assessment of chromosomes is carried out. Useful in the diagnosis of chromosomal disorders with numerical abnormalities (trisomy 21, trisomy 18, trisomy 13, Turner syndrome—45XO)

2. **Fluorescent *in situ* hybridization (FISH):** Provides specific localization of genes on chromosomes. Specific probes (fluorescently labeled) are used to bind a region of interest on the chromosome. Useful in diagnosis of trisomies and microdeletion syndromes, e.g. diGeorge syndrome.

3. **Comparative genomic hybridization (CGH):** This is a special FISH technique, useful in the diagnosis of all the genomic imbalances. Array CGH, a more advanced technique, is used to scan the genome for gains or losses of chromosomal material. This is used to diagnose patients with developmental delay/mental retardation and/or multiple congenital anomalies.

4. **Sanger sequencing:** Gold standard to diagnose genetic disorders with abnormal DNA sequence/mutations. This technique is useful to diagnose mutations in patients with PID with a known gene. For exmaple, in a case of X-linked agammaglobulinemia, the sequencing of the BTK gene by the Sanger method will provide the diagnosis.

5. **Next generation sequencing (NGS):** The term NGS is used to describe highly parallel or high-output sequencing methods. It is a type of DNA sequencing technology that uses parallel sequencing of multiple small fragments of DNA to determine the sequence. In contrast to Sanger sequencing, the speed of sequencing and amounts of DNA sequence data generated with NGS, are exponentially greater and are produced at reduced costs.

In other words, thousands of genes can be sequenced simultaneously in a short span. This would be a more cost-effective approach compared to Sanger sequencing when sequencing of multiple genes is needed to arrive at a diagnosis.

Sanger vs NGS

While Sanger sequencing of the suspected gene is likely to yield the genetic diagnosis, it is not cost-effective to perform Sanger sequencing of several hundred genes to determine the diagnosis in a suspected case of PID. It would be extremely laborious and time-consuming as well! Let's consider a child with severe combined immune deficiency (SCID). More than a dozen genes have been implicated in the causation of SCID and with ongoing research, new genes are constantly being added! Performing Sanger sequencing of all these genes would be a tedious task, consuming a lot of time and money. Next generation sequencing (NGS), on the other hand, can simultaneously sequence all these genes and provide results in a short span of time, at a much cheaper cost.

Several laboratories now provide genetic testing by NGS and offer targeted panels for PID. However, in the absence of adequate clinical information, performing NGS in a random fashion would be a futile exercise. Performing basic immunological tests and arriving at a possible differential diagnosis is a pre-requisite before one orders a genetic test.

What can NGS miss?

Large deletions and complex mutations.

Note: The current gold standard method for chromosomal microdeletions and microduplications analysis is array CGH.

Let us discuss a few cases.

Case 1

A 3 year-old boy presented with recurrent pneumonia and draining ears. Family history was significant. This family had lost two boys at the age of 9 and 6, respectively. Both the boys had recurrent infections and succumbed to their illness. They also had a girl child who was doing fine.

Investigations: All the immunoglobulins were low (panhypogammaglobulinemia) and B cells were absent.

Clinical diagnosis: X-linked agammaglobulinemia (XLA) (refer Chapter 28 for more details on XLA)

XLA is due to a defect in the Bruton tyrosine kinase (BTK) gene.

Hence, one can look for a mutation in the BTK gene by Sanger sequencing. However, several genes are implicated in causing agammaglobulinemia (AR inheritance). Hence, NGS could be performed that will be able to diagnose mutations in BTK and other genes as well.

Case 2

A 4-month-old girl presented with persistent oral thrush and failure to thrive. She had an episode of pneumonia and was hospitalized.

Investigations
+ HIV negative.

Lymphocyte subsets
+ CD3–2% (50–70%)
+ CD19–91% (10–15%)
+ CD56–3% (5–10%)

Markedly reduced T cells in this setting confirm a diagnosis of **severe combined immune deficiency (SCID).**

Which genetic testing platform would you choose? NGS or Sanger sequencing?

As highlighted previously, several genes are implicated in the causation of SCID and hence NGS study (targeted clinical exome/whole exome) that covers all the genes involved in SCID must be performed.

Clinical exome was ordered by NGS—homozygous pathogenic mutation was identified in exon 2 of the JAK3 gene.

Final diagnosis: SCID due to JAK3 gene mutation (AR inheritance).

This was further confirmed by Sanger sequencing. Parents were counselled and Sanger sequencing was carried out in both the parents targeting exon 2 of the JAK3 gene. Both had the same mutation in the heterozygous state, confirming they are carriers.

Case 3

A 2-year-old boy was admitted with severe pneumonia. Past history was significant. He was hospitalized twice in the first year of life, and had been treated for sepsis with IV antibiotics. He also had mild developmental delay and had hypocalcemic seizures at 6 months of age.

In view of recurrent infections, a possibility of immune deficiency was considered. Basic immunological screen (immunoglobulins, lymphocyte subsets) was normal.

Genetic testing by NGS was ordered.

Result: No mutation identified.

Case was reviewed again:

a. Hypocalcemia: Further investigations showed low parathyroid hormone levels, confirming hypoparathyroidism.

b. Hypoparathyroidism + Developmental delay + Recurrent infections— A possibility of DiGeorge syndrome was considered

FISH study for DiGeorge syndrome was asked for.

Result: 22q11.2 deleted, suggestive of DiGeorge syndrome.

Message

1. A detailed assessment of the clinical case and arriving at a few differential diagnoses is very important before one orders a genetic test.

2. Choosing the right platform for genetic testing is very crucial in arriving at an appropriate diagnosis. In case 3, while a FISH study picked up the diagnosis of DiGeorge syndrome, NGS study was not warranted. NGS is a costly test and most laboratories often need 4–6 weeks for reporting. It must be used judiciously.

Remember

Single gene diseases→NGS followed by Sanger sequencing.
Microdeletions/syndromes →Array CGH/FISH
(These tests are not mutually exclusive and are complementary).

Note:
✦ Written informed consent must be taken before performing a genetic test.
✦ Pre-test and post-test genetic counselling must be offered.

Did you know?
The Human Genome Project is the world's largest collaborative biological project which extended for 13 years (1990–2003). It involved mapping of all the genes of human genome.

SUGGESTED READING

1. Bisgin A, Boga I, Yilmaz M, Bingol G, Altintas D. The Utility of Next-Generation Sequencing for Primary Immunodeficiency Disorders: Experience from a Clinical Diagnostic Laboratory. *Biomed Res Int*. 2018; 2018:9647253.

2. Chi ZH, Wei W, Bu DF, Li HH, Ding F, Zhu P. Targeted high-throughput sequencing technique for the molecular diagnosis of primary immunodeficiency disorders. *Medicine (Baltimore)*. 2018; 97(40):e12695.

3. Heimall J. Now Is the Time to Use Molecular Gene Testing for the Diagnosis of Primary Immune Deficiencies. *J Allergy Clin Immunol Pract*. 2019; 7(3):833–838.

Principles of Treatment in Primary Immune Deficiency

Three major forms of treatment in PIDs:
1. Hematopoietic stem cell transplant (HSCT)/Bone marrow transplant (BMT)
2. Immunoglobulin replacement
3. Antimicrobial prophylaxis

HSCT/BMT

BMT is curative in the majority of PIDs and is the treatment of choice for severe forms of PID.

SCID is a medical emergency and is 100% fatal in the absence of BMT. Children with SCID, if transplanted early, before they develop serious infections, can be cured with a success rate >90%! Hence early diagnosis and referral to a center with expertise in the management of these cases are essential.

Some of the common PIDs where BMT is curative:
1. Severe combined immune deficiency
2. Chronic granulomatous disease
3. Leukocyte adhesion deficiency
4. Wiskott-Aldrich syndrome
5. Severe congenital neutropenia
6. X-linked hyper-IgM syndrome (due to CD40L defect)
7. Primary HLH (hemophagocytic lymphohistiocytosis)

8. Severe forms of MSMD (Mendelian susceptibility to mycobacterial disease)

A wide variety of PIDs can be treated with BMT. With a better understanding of these diseases and improvement in the outcomes of BMT, many diseases have now been considered as candidates for BMT.

Immunoglobulin (Ig) Replacement Therapy

Children and adults with B cell defects must be treated with Ig replacement.

Examples
+ X-linked agammaglobulinemia (XLA)
+ Common variable immune deficiency (CVID)
+ Hyper-IgM syndrome

Note: Patients with dysgammaglobulinemia can also be treated with replacement IVIg therapy, e.g. Wiskott-Aldrich syndrome (WAS).

Dosage: Intravenous immunoglobulin (IVIg) 400 mg/kg/month (dose can be adjusted to maintain trough IgG levels >500 mg/dl). Higher doses are needed in patients with bronchiectasis.

Duration: Lifelong in the case of XLA and CVID. Patients with WAS are treated with monthly IVIg infusions until they receive a bone marrow transplant.

It is heartening to note that several state governments across India are now providing IVIg free of cost to several patients with PID.

Note
1. During an inter-current infection, 1 g/kg of IVIg may be given to tide-over the crisis.
2. Children with XLA, when treated with regular IVIg infusions lead a normal life and grow to become productive citizens.
3. Subcutaneous immunoglobulins are regularly being administered in many of the Western countries, however, such preparations are not yet available in India (and maybe launched into the market soon).

Antimicrobial Prophylaxis

This would be useful in the following settings.

1. Milder forms of PIDs can be managed with antibiotic prophylaxis, e.g. patients with AD-hyper IgE syndrome have a remarkable reduction in the risk of infections on cotrimoxazole prophylaxis. However, such prophylaxis needs to be continued indefinitely.

2. Antimicrobial prophylaxis may be used as a bridge while preparing patients for BMT in certain PIDs, e.g. chronic granulomatous disease.

Type of prophylaxis depends on the underlying PID.

A. **Chronic granulomatous disease**
   + Cotrimoxazole + Itraconazole (Antibacterial + Antifungal) {Cotrimoxazole 5 mg/kg/day—trimethoprim dose, itraconazole 100 mg (<50 kg), 200 mg (>50 kg) once daily}

B. **Hyper-IgM syndrome (X-linked)**
   + Cotrimoxazole + Itraconazole (+ IVIg replacement therapy)

C. **Hyper-IgE syndrome (AD)**
   + Cotrimoxazole or penicillin

D. **IgG subclass deficiency**
   + Cotrimoxazole

Did you know?

What's a chimera?

+ A fire-breathing female monster with a lion's head, a goat's body, and a serpent's tail (as per Greek mythology).

+ Following a bone marrow transplant, a patient would have a mixture of donor and host stem cells. The hematopoietic system is thereby a mixture of two individuals!

A REAL CHIMERA!

SUGGESTED READING

1. Albin S, Cunningham-Rundles C. An update on the use of immunoglobulin for the treatment of immunodeficiency disorders. *Immunotherapy*. 2014; 6(10):1113–1126. doi:10.2217/imt.14.67

2. Azizi G, Ziaee V, Tavakol M, et al. Approach to the Management of Autoimmunity in Primary Immunodeficiency. *Scand J Immunol*. 2017; 85(1):13–29.

3. Bonagura VR. Using intravenous immunoglobulin (IVIG) to treat patients with primary immune deficiency disease. *J Clin Immunol*. 2013; 33 Suppl 2:S90–S94.

4. Castagnoli R, Delmonte OM, Calzoni E, Notarangelo LD. Hematopoietic Stem Cell Transplantation in Primary Immunodeficiency Diseases: Current Status and Future Perspectives. *Front Pediatr*. 2019; 7:295.

5. Rivers L, Gaspar HB. Severe combined immunodeficiency: recent developments and guidance on clinical management. *Arch Dis Child*. 2015; 100(7):667–672.

When is an Immune Deficiency a Medical Emergency?

Children with severe combined immune deficiency present in infancy with failure to thrive, recurrent pneumonia, diarrhea, oral thrush and other opportunistic infections (CMV retinitis, disseminated atypical mycobacterial infection, etc.). This condition is universally fatal and the majority of children would die before the age of 2. This condition warrants an urgent bone marrow transplant. Hence, **SCID is a medical emergency** (refer Chapters 14 and 28 for details on SCID).

In the Western and developed world, screening for SCID is a part of the newborn screening program (TREC assay is the screening test used). These children are thereby diagnosed within the first few weeks of life, even before they acquire any serious infection and they undergo BMT with a success rate >93%. On the contrary, in our set-up, the majority of children with SCID are diagnosed after they acquire an infection. Any further delay in the institution of appropriate care would prove fatal in these cases! Hence these children must be urgently referred to centers with experience in the management of these diseases.

Some important facts on SCID:
1. Persistent lymphopenia in an infant is a strong clue towards underlying SCID.
2. Persistent oral thrush and failure to thrive in an infant warrant an evaluation for possible SCID.
3. History of sibling deaths in early infancy could be a pointer. The presence of such family history must make one think of SCID in the index child, even if the infant appears healthy.

4. Urgent referral of suspected SCID to appropriate centers is necessary to provide optimal care and outcome.

5. One must always offer genetic testing to babies with SCID, even if they are critically ill. This would help in establishing the molecular diagnosis and providing an antenatal diagnosis in the subsequent pregnancy.

Did you know?

Nude SCID:

Mutation in FOXN1 gene, results in thymic agenesis and alopecia totalis.

Omenn syndrome:

SCID where T cells are present! Presents in early infancy with diffuse erythroderma, lymphadenopathy and organomegaly, eosinophilia and high IgE.

SUGGESTED READING

1. Delmonte OM, Schuetz C, Notarangelo LD. RAG Deficiency: Two Genes, Many Diseases. *J Clin Immunol*. 2018; 38(6):646–655.

2. Kato M, Kimura H, Seki M, et al. Omenn syndrome—review of several phenotypes of Omenn syndrome and RAG1/RAG2 mutations in Japan. *Allergol Int*. 2006; 55(2):115–119.

3. Rota IA, Dhalla F. FOXN1 deficient nude severe combined immunodeficiency. *Orphanet J Rare Dis*. 2017; 12(1):6.

Vaccination in Primary Immune Deficiency

Patients with PID may not be able to mount a normal response to vaccines, moreover, children with certain PIDs are at risk for serious complications to live vaccines (e.g. disseminated BCG infection in children with SCID). Children with complement defects are at risk for infections with encapsulated bacteria and thereby, vaccinations that protect against such bacteria must be administered in these patients.

A. **B cell defects, e.g. XLA, CVID**
   - Live vaccines—contraindicated (especially, oral polio vaccine)
   - Killed vaccines—no benefit (these children are on regular IVIg infusions)
   - Killed influenza vaccine to be given yearly

B. **T cell defects, e.g. SCID**
   - All vaccinations are contraindicated. BCG vaccine must be avoided in a newborn if the previous child in the family had been diagnosed to/suspected to have SCID until immunological tests rule out SCID in the index baby.

C. **Chronic granulomatous disease**
   - BCG vaccine is contraindicated.
   - Other vaccines can be given.

D. **Complement deficiency**
   - Pneumococcal, meningococcal, typhoid vaccines must be given.
   - All routine vaccines can be given.

Did you know?

Oral polio vaccine must be avoided in all the family members and close contacts of patients with T and B cell defects (SCID, CID and immunoglobulin deficiency).

SUGGESTED READING

Eibl MM, Wolf HM. Vaccination in patients with primary immune deficiency, secondary immune deficiency and autoimmunity with immune regulatory abnormalities. *Immunotherapy*. 2015; 7(12):1273–1292.

Immunology Tests: EDTA Sample? Heparinized Sample? Serum?

Medical residents and busy pediatricians often find it difficult to recall which samples need to be sent for immunological and genetic tests. Some of the samples are time-critical and others need a healthy control to match with, while the tests are performed. It would be prudent to understand what samples need to be sent to the laboratory before one bleeds the child. After all, sampling a small child is never an easy task!

For easy reference, I have tabulated various investigations and the relevant samples to be sent. Please note that certain samples need to be fresh (<24-hour transit between sampling and processing in the lab). For example, lymphocyte subsets (T cell, B cell, NK cell) assessment would not yield any meaningful result, if the sample is not processed in time, as cells would degenerate and you would get falsely low counts.

Table 25.1: Immunological tests—A quick guide

Test	Testing platform	Vacutainer	Healthy control	Comments
Immunoglobulins (IgG, IgA, IgM)	Nephelometry/ turbidimetry	Plain vacutainer (serum)	Not needed	If delay in transport, store at 2–8°C.
Immunoglobulin IgE	ELISA	Plain vacutainer	Not needed	If delay in transport, store at 2–8°C.

Contd.

Table 25.1: Immunological tests—A quick guide *(Contd.)*

Test	Testing platform	Vacutainer	Healthy control	Comments
Lymphocyte subsets (T cell, B cell, NK cells)	Flow cytometry	EDTA	Not needed	To be processed within 24–48 hrs.
CD4 and CD8 counts	Flow cytometry	EDTA	Not needed	To be processed within 24–48 hrs.
NBT	Microscopy	Sodium heparin	Needed	To be processed within 24 hrs.
DHR	Flow cytometry	Sodium heparin	Needed	To be processed within 24 hrs.
CD18, CD11	Flow cytometry	Sodium heparin	Needed	Testing for suspected LAD.
Genetic testing (whole exome sequencing)	NGS	EDTA	Not needed	If delay in transport, store at 2–8°C.

LAD—leukocyte adhesion deficiency, NGS—next generation sequencing

> **Did you know?**
> + DHR will have two peaks (mosaic pattern) in female carriers of X-linked CGD (mothers).
> + Do not use mother (or family members) as controls, while performing a DHR test.

Algorithms for Quick Reference

(A) Children with recurrent pneumonia/ear infections/diarrhea/failure to thrive
↓
CBC
↓
Lymphopenia (ALC < 3000/mm^3 in infants)
↓
Think of SCID (severe combined immune deficiency)
↓
Look for thymus in chest radiograph/ultrasound neck;
order serum immunoglobulins and lymphocyte subsets (T, B and NK cell counts)
↓
Hypogammaglobulinemia and low T cell counts
↓
Consistent with diagnosis of **SCID**
↓
Store EDTA sample for genetic testing and urgent referral for BMT

(B) Recurrent pneumonia/ear infections in a boy child
↓
Clinical examination shows absent tonsils and lymph nodes;
immunoglobulin assay shows low IgG, IgA and IgM
↓
Lymphocyte subsets (T, B and NK cell counts)
↓
B cell counts reduced (<2%)
↓
Likely diagnosis—**X-linked agammaglobulinemia**
↓
BTK protein expression by flow cytometry AND genetic testing
↓
Treatment—IVIg 400 mg/kg/month

(C) Adolescents/adults presenting with recurrent pneumonia/ear
infections/sinusitis/diarrhea
↓
Order immunoglobulins IgG, IgA and IgM
↓
low IgG AND low IgA/IgM
↓
Lymphocyte subsets (T, B and NK cell counts)—normal
↓
Likely diagnosis—**common variable immune deficiency**
↓
B cell immunophenotyping, assess vaccine responses, hemagglutinin titres
(anti-A and anti-B titres)
↓
Treatment—IVIg 400 mg/kg/month

(D) Recurrent suppurative infections (lymphadenitis/lung or liver abscess/osteomyelitis)
↓
CBC shows neutrophilia, thrombocytosis;
immunoglobulins—high IgG
↓
Order NBT and DHR
↓
Abnormal NBT and DHR
↓
Likely diagnosis—**chronic granulomatous disease**
↓
Genetic testing
↓
Start co-trimoxazole and itraconazole prophylaxis and prepare for BMT

(E) Boy with recurrent infections + Eczema
↓
Persistent thrombocytopenia
↓
Think of **Wiskott-Aldrich syndrome** (WAS)
↓
Look for mean platelet volume (MPV)
"Low MPV is a strong pointer towards WAS"
↓
High IgE is seen in most of the patients
↓
WASP expression by flow cytometry AND genetic testing
↓
Treatment—IVIg 400 mg/kg/month + Co-trimoxazole prophylaxis AND prepare for BMT

(F) Recurrent infections + History of delay in cord fall/omphalitis
↓
Persistent neutrophilia
↓
Suspect **leucocyte adhesion deficiency** (LAD)
↓
CD18 and CD11a assay by flow cytometry
↓
Reduced CD18/CD11 expression—consistent with diagnosis of LAD
↓
Genetic testing
↓
Treatment—cotrimoxazole + itraconazole prophylaxis and
prepare for BMT in case of severe LAD (CD18 <1%)

(G) Recurrent infections in infancy
↓
CBC shows persistent neutropenia (ANC <1500/mm^3)
↓
Bone marrow exam—arrest in myeloid differentiation
↓
Likely diagnosis—**severe congenital neutropenia**
↓
Genetic testing
↓
Treatment—start G-CSF therapy and consider BMT if refractory to G-CSF therapy.

Age-specific Norms for Immunoglobulins and Lymphocyte Subsets

One must always look at the age norms while interpreting the results of immunoglobulin assay and lymphocyte subsets. Many labs provide only adult norms which are irrelevant to the pediatric population. The following tables can be used as a reference when immunological tests are performed.

Reference (Quoted by NELSON textbook of Pediatrics)

Meites S, editor: Pediatric clinical chemistry, reference (normal) values, ed 3, Washington, DC, 1989, American Association for Clinical Chemistry.

Table 27.1: Age norms for serum immunoglobulins	
IgG	**mg/dl**
Cord blood	636–1,606
1 mo	251–906
2–4 mo	176–601
5–12 mo	172–1,069
1–5 yr	345–1,236
6–10 yr	608–1,572
Adult	639–1,349

Contd.

Table 27.1: Age norms for serum immunoglobulins (*Contd.*)

IgA	mg/dl
Cord blood	1.4–3.6
1–3 mo	1.3–53
4–6 mo	4.4–84
7 mo–1 yr	11–106
2–5 yr	14–159
6–10 yr	33–236
Adult	70–312
IgM	**mg/dl**
Cord blood	6.3–25
1–4 mo	17–105
5–9 mo	33–126
10 mo–1 yr	41–173
2–8 yr	43–207
9–10 yr	52–242
Adult	56–352

Indian study by Narula G, et al. has produced the following age norms for serum immunoglobulins.

Table 27.2: Age norms for serum immunoglobulins			
Age	**IgG (mg/dl)**	**IgM (mg/dl)**	**IgA (mg/dl)**
Cord blood	156–1800	0–44	0.5–7.3
0–6 months	309–1573	3.7–89	7.8–57.8
7–12 months	170–1053	6–138	22–98
13–36 months	130–2040	78–658	46–158
37–60 months	796–2178	85–249	83.5–239

[**Reference:** Narula G, Khodaiji S, Bableshwar A, Bindra MS. Age-related reference intervals for immunoglobulin levels and lymphocyte subsets in Indian children. *Indian J Pathol Microbiol.* 2017 Jul–Sep; 60(3):360–364]

Table 27.3: Age-wise norms for lymphocyte subsets (in cells/mm³)					
Age	**CD4**	**CD8**	**CD3**	**CD19**	**CD16/56**
Cord blood	2209–3205	312–1360	3100–5200	61–2447	-
0–6 months	1516–4348	970–2118	1767–5495	860–2215	5.8–35
7–12 months	1056–3799	541–2807	1278–4710	25–1809	7.8–8.9
13–36 months	1113–2946	523–2015	1222–3790	88–1576	54.5–261.5
37–60 months	839–3115	749–1997	1368–3812	56–1697	53–1160

[**Reference:** Narula G, Khodaiji S, Bableshwar A, Bindra MS. Age-related reference intervals for immunoglobulin levels and lymphocyte subsets in Indian children. Indian *J Pathol Microbiol.* 2017 Jul–Sep; 60(3):360–364]

Table 27.4: Percentages of peripheral blood lymphocytes in healthy children

Subset	0–3 mo	3–6 mo	6–12 mo	1–2 yr	2–6 yr	6–12 yr	12–18 yr
CD3	73 (53–84)	66 (51–77)	65 (49–76)	65 (53–75)	66 (56–75)	69 (60–76)	73 (56–84)
CD19	15 (06–32)	25 (11–41)	24 (14–37)	25 (16–35)	21 (14–33)	18 (13–27)	14 (06–23)
CD16/56	8 (04–18)	6 (03–14)	7 (03–15)	7 (03–15)	9 (04–17)	9 (04–17)	9 (03–22)
CD4	52 (35–64)	46 (35–56)	46 (31–56)	41 (32–51)	38 (28–47)	37 (31–47)	41 (31–52)
CD8	18 (12–28)	16 (12–23)	17 (12–24)	20 (14–30)	23 (16–30)	25 (18–35)	26 (18–35)

[Reference: Shearer WT, Rosenblatt HM, Gelman RS, et al. Lymphocyte subsets in healthy children from birth through 18 years of age: The Pediatric AIDS Clinical Trials Group P1009 study. *J Allergy Clin Immunol.* 2003; 112(5):973–980]

Table 27.5: Subset counts of peripheral blood lymphocytes in healthy children ($\times 10^3/mm^3$)

Subset	0–3 mo	3–6 mo	6–12 mo	1–2 yr	2–6 yr	6–12 yr	12–18 yr
WBC	10.60 (7.20–18.00)	9.20 (6.70–14.00)	9.10 (6.40–13.00)	8.80 (6.40–12.00)	7.10 (5.20–11.00)	6.50 (4.40–9.50)	6.00 (4.40–8.10)
Lympho-cytes	5.40 (3.40–7.60)	6.30 (3.90–9.00)	5.90 (3.40–9.00)	5.50 (3.60–8.90)	3.60 (2.30–5.40)	2.70 (1.90–3.70)	2.20 (1.40–3.30)
CD3	3.68 (2.50–5.50)	3.93 (2.50–5.60)	3.93 (1.90–5.90)	3.55 (2.10–6.20)	2.39 (1.40–3.70)	1.82 (1.20–2.60)	1.48 (1.00–2.20)

Contd.

Table 27.5: Subset counts of peripheral blood lymphocytes in healthy children (× 10³/mm³) (*Contd.*)

Subset	0–3 mo	3–6 mo	6–12 mo	1–2 yr	2–6 yr	6–12 yr	12–18 yr
CD19	0.73 (0.30–2.00)	1.55 (0.43–3.00)	1.52 (0.61–2.60)	1.31 (0.72–2.60)	0.75 (0.39–1.40)	0.48 (0.27–0.86)	0.30 (0.11–0.57)
CD 16/56	0.42 (0.17–1.10)	0.42 (0.17–0.83)	0.40 (0.16–0.95)	0.36 (0.18–0.92)	0.30 (0.13–0.72)	0.23 (0.10–0.48)	0.19 (0.07–0.48)
CD4	2.61 (1.60–4.00)	2.85 (1.80–4.00)	2.67 (1.40–4.30)	2.16 (1.30–3.40)	1.38 (0.70–2.20)	0.98 (0.65–1.50)	0.84 (0.53–1.30)
CD8	0.98 (0.56–1.70)	1.05 (0.59–1.60)	1.04 (0.50–1.70)	1.04 (0.62–2.00)	0.84 (0.49–1.30)	0.68 (0.37–1.10)	0.53 (0.33–0.92)

[**Reference:** Shearer WT, Rosenblatt HM, Gelman RS, et al. Lymphocyte subsets in healthy children from birth through 18 years of age: The Pediatric AIDS Clinical Trials Group P1009 study. *J Allergy Clin Immunol*. 2003; 112(5):973–980]

Commonly Diagnosed Immune Deficiencies: A Quick Review

B Cell Disorders/Humoral Defects

Humoral defects contribute to around 50% of all the PIDs. A brief note on some of the commonly diagnosed humoral immune deficiencies will be provided here.

X-linked Agammaglobulinemia

(Previously called 'Bruton agammaglobulinemia')

Etiology: Mutation in Bruton tyrosine kinase (BTK) gene located on X-chromosome.

Pathogenesis: Arrest in B cell development during the pro-B stage, resulting in severe B cell lymphopenia, panhypogammaglobulinemia and paucity of secondary lymphoid organs.

Clinical presentation: Recurrent infections in affected boys. Onset >6 months of age.

+ **Common infections:** Sinusitis, otitis media, pneumonia (complication—bronchiectasis).
+ **Other issues:** Meningitis, enteroviral encephalitis, arthritis (caused by *Mycoplasma* and *Ureaplasma*)
+ **Organisms**: *S. pneumonia, H. influenza, E. coli, S. aureus, Klebsiella, Giardia, Enterovirus.*

Immunological phenotype: Low IgG, IgA, and IgM. Absent B cells.

Treatment: IVIg 400 mg/kg/month for life.

IgA Deficiency

+ IgA deficiency—Serum IgA < –2SD for age.
+ Selective IgA deficiency—IgA <7 mg/dl.

Etiology: The basic defect is unknown. In certain families, IgA deficiency is noted in multiple members in successive generations and hence an autosomal dominant pattern of inheritance is suspected.

Drugs causing IgA deficiency: Phenytoin, D-penicillamine, gold, and sulphasalazine.

Clinical presentation: Though IgA deficiency is common in certain populations, it is a mild immune deficiency and patients present with recurrent sino-pulmonary infections.

Common infections: Sinusitis, otitis media, chronic diarrhea (related to giardiasis).
Autoimmune disorders are increased in patients with IgA deficiency.

> **Note:** Children presenting with serious infections and low IgA levels (and normal IgG) must be investigated for IgG2 subclass deficiency. Children with IgA deficiency must be followed up as some of them may evolve into CVID (common variable immune deficiency).

Common Variable Immunodeficiency (CVID)

+ Most common symptomatic immune deficiency in adults.
+ Syndrome characterized by low immunoglobulins and normal B cells.

Etiology: Most patients do not have an identified genetic defect. Underlying genetic defect with autosomal recessive or dominant inheritance—identified in 10% cases. Genes—ICOS, BAFF-R, CD19, CD20, CD21, CD81, TACI, etc.

Pathogenesis: Though B cells are present in normal numbers they fail to differentiate into antibody-producing plasma cells.

Clinical presentation: Onset in adolescents and adults. It is prudent to remember that a majority of patients with CVID would first present to adult physicians, gastroenterologists, and pulmonologists.

Common infections: Sinusitis, otitis media, pneumonia, diarrhea.

✦ Recurrent pneumonia leads to bronchiectasis.

✦ Increased predisposition to autoimmune disorders—autoimmune hemolytic anemia, immune thrombocytopenia, arthritis, alopecia areata, pernicious anemia.

✦ Increased risk of lymphoma and gastric carcinoma.

✦ Non-caseating granulomas affecting lung, liver, spleen, and skin can be seen.

Organisms: *S. pneumonia, H. influenza, Mycoplasma, Giardia, Norovirus,* etc.

Diagnosis: Recurrent infections/autoimmunity and **low IgG** and low IgA or low IgM and exclusion of other causes of hypogammaglobulinemia.

Increased risk of malignancies: Non-Hodgkin lymphoma, gastric carcinoma.

Immunological phenotype: Hypogammaglobulinemia with normal B cells.

Treatment: IVIg 400 mg/kg/month for life.

IgG2 Subclass Deficiency

✦ Four IgG subclasses—IgG1, IgG2, IgG3, and IgG4.

✦ IgG2 protects against polysaccharides (encapsulated bacteria).

Etiology: Unknown

Clinical presentation: Recurrent infections with encapsulated bacteria (*S. pneumonia, H. influenza,* etc.).

Diagnosis: Total IgG is normal or elevated (due to compensatory increase in other IgG subclasses). Low IgG2 levels for age.

Clinically significant IgG2 deficiency = IgG2 subclass deficiency + Poor vaccine response

Only clinically significant IgG2 deficiency warrants treatment.

Treatment: Antibiotic prophylaxis (cotrimoxazole), vaccination (pneumo-coccal conjugate vaccine followed by PPSV23). Despite these measures, if there are ongoing infections, consider IVIg 400 mg/kg/month.

Note: Patients with IgA deficiency and significant infections must be investigated for IgG2 deficiency.

Hyper-IgM Syndrome

✦ Class switch disorders.

✦ Characterized by normal or high IgM in presence of low IgG and IgA.

✦ Five types: Most common type—type 1 hyper-IgM syndrome (X-linked) caused by CD40—ligand deficiency.

Etiology: Defect in class switch.

Pathogenesis: Please note the Fig. 28.1.

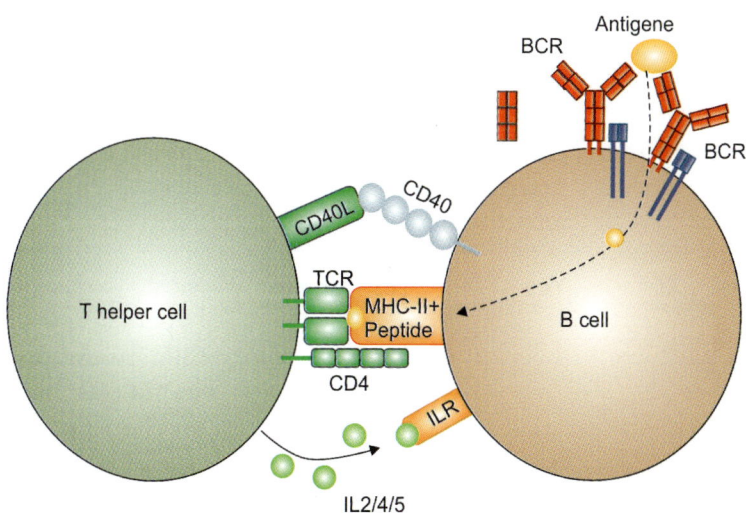

(Author attribute: By Altaileopard - Own work, Public Domain, https://commons.wikimedia.org/w/index.php?curid = 12193556)

Fig. 28.1: Pathogenesis of Hyper-IgM syndrome

B cells produce IgM in response to an antigen (infection). Later, T and B cells interact with each other in lymph nodes and as a result, B cells start producing other classes of immunoglobulins (IgG, IgA or IgE). B cells express CD40 and activated T cells express CD40 ligand. Interaction between CD40 and CD40L is crucial for class switching and hence deficiency of CD40 or CD40L would result in class switch defect. B cells in these patients (with deficiency of CD40L or CD40) only produce IgM and with every infection, IgM levels keep rising; thereby causing hyper-IgM syndrome.

Note: 50% of patients with hyper-IgM syndrome have normal IgM levels and hence the term 'hyper-IgM syndrome' is a misnomer. All patients have low IgG, IgA, and IgE.

Clinical presentation: Recurrent infections from early childhood—recurrent pneumonia, ear infections and diarrhea. Patients with X-linked hyper-IgM syndrome (defect in CD40L) can present with P*pneumocystis jirovecii* pneumonia in infancy. They are predisposed to cryptosporidiosis and this may result in biliary cirrhosis. Increased predisposition to biliary tumors in the second and third decade of life has been noted. The following table (Table 28.1) provides important information on various types of hyper-IgM syndrome.

Table 28.1: Overview of the different types of hyper-IgM syndrome

Type	Defect	Inheritance	Opportunistic infections	IVIg	HSCT	Salient features
1.	CD40L	XL	Yes	Yes	Yes	Most common type of hyper-IgM syndrome. PJP pneumonia, cryptosporidiosis, biliary cirrhosis and hepatic tumors
2.	AICDA	AR	No	Yes	No	Enlarged lymph nodes with giant germinal centres
3.	CD40	AR	Yes	Yes	Yes	Opportunistic infections can occur
4.	Not known	AR	No	Yes	No	Rare
5.	UNG	AR	No	Yes	No	Rare (few case reports)

(CD40L:CD40 ligand, AICDA: Activation-induced Cytidine Deaminase, UNG—Uracil DNA Glycosylase, PJP—*Pneumocystis jirovecii pneumonia*, XL—X-linked, AR—autosomal recessive)

Immunological phenotype: Normal or high IgM, low IgG, and IgA and IgE. Normal B cell counts. Reduced memory B cells.

Treatment: Monthly IVIg, cotrimoxazole and itraconazole prophylaxis. Type 1 and 3 warrant a BMT.

Combined Defects

As T cell help is crucial for B cell function, T cell defects often result in B cell dysfunction. These disorders are called combined defects. Let us discuss a few of them.

  A. SCID—Severe combined immune deficiency
  B. CID—Combined immune deficiency

SCID

The most severe form of immune deficiency characterized by absent T cells.

Etiology: More than a dozen genes have been implicated in the causation.

Pathogenesis: Defect in the development of T cells. Small or absent thymus noted in the majority.

Clinical presentation: Present in early infancy with pneumonia, diarrhea, oral thrush and failure to thrive. Universally fatal in the absence of a bone marrow transplant.

Diagnosis: The presence of lymphopenia (ALC <3000/mm^3) in infants is a clue to underlying SCID.
  Lymphocyte subset analysis shows absent T cells (CD^3 < 20% of lymphocytes).
  Absolute CD3 < 300/mm^3 is diagnostic.

Types: X-linked SCID, caused by a mutation in the IL2RG gene; AR- SCID can be caused by mutations in several genes—ADA, JAK3, RAG1, RAG2, etc.
  Immunological phenotype may suggest the underlying genetic defect (Table 28.2).

Table 28.2: Genetic defect	
Immunological phenotype	*Genetic defect*
T-B+NK-	IL2RG, JAK3
T-B-NK-	ADA, PNP
T-B-NK+	RAG1, RAG2, DNA ligase IV, Cernunnos, Artemis (DCLRE1C)
T-B+NK+	IL7Ra

Treatment: Bone marrow transplant. SCID is a medical emergency and an urgent BMT is warranted in this setting.

Combined Immune Defects (CID)

A group of disorders with defect in T-cell number or function. These are not as severe as SCID and hence these children usually survive beyond 2 years of age.

When do you suspect CID?

Children presenting with opportunistic infections (viral/fungal, etc.) and surviving beyond the age of 2.

Many of them have associated autoimmunity and granulomatous manifestations (granulomas in gut, liver, lymph nodes, lungs).

Persistent lymphopenia must raise a suspicion of CID in a patient with recurrent/unusual infections.

Examples:
+ DOCK8 deficiency.
+ CTLA-4 haploinsufficiency (CHAI).
+ Activated phosphokinase delta syndrome (APDS).

Diagnosis
+ Presence of lymphopenia may be a clue.
+ Reduced T-cell counts may be noted.
+ Hypogammaglobulinemia.

Genetic testing: Confirms the diagnosis.

Syndromes with Immune Deficiency

DiGeorge Syndrome

Etiology: 22q11.2 microdeletion

Pathogenesis: Defective development of third and fourth pharyngeal pouches

Clinical features: Congenital heart defect, hypoparathyroidism resulting in hypocalcemia, abnormal facies, immune deficiency.

Immune deficiency in DiGeorge syndrome

Immune deficiency is variable and children with DiGeorge syndrome can be classified into

a. Partial DiGeorge has a small thymus: Naïve T cells less than 10th percentile for age but more than $50/mm^3$.
b. Complete DiGeorge is characterized by Athymia (absent thymus): Naive CD3 T cells $<50/mm^3$ or less than 5% of total T cells.

Only a small proportion of patients with DiGeorge syndrome have the complete form. This disease is universally fatal by the age of 2. Hence, an early diagnosis and thymic transplant are warranted in infants with complete DiGeorge syndrome.

Diagnosis: Microarray for 22q11.2 microdeletion (FISH study).

Immunological evaluation: All children with DiGeorge syndrome must be investigated for serum immunoglobulins, lymphocyte subsets (CD3, CD4, CD8, CD19 and CD56) and naïve T cells. Children with absent naïve T cells must be counselled for thymic transplant.

Treatment: Multidisciplinary management—cardiologist, endocrinologist and immunologist must be involved.

Wiskott-Aldrich Syndrome (WAS)

Triad of recurrent infections, eczema, and low platelets.

Etiology: X-linked recessive disorder. Mutation in the WASP gene, resulting in loss of expression or function of WAS protein.

Pathogenesis: WAS protein (WASP) is selectively expressed in the hematopoietic system and involved in the cytoskeletal-organizing complex and the maturation, activation, and transport of blood elements. WASP is essential for the formation of immunological synapses (cell-cell contacts for immunological response). A deficiency in WASP results in defective development of platelets (resulting in thrombocytopenia) and a defect in cellular and humoral immunity resulting in a combined immune deficiency.

Clinical presentation

  a. Recurrent infections from early childhood—pneumonia, ear infections, diarrhea, meningitis.
  b. Passage of blood in motions—colitis.
  c. Increased risk of lymphoid malignancies in the second decade of life.
  d. Persistent thrombocytopenia from birth.
  e. Eosinophilia may be present.

Diagnosis

✦ In every boy with persistent thrombocytopenia, one must look at mean platelet volume (MPV).

✦ Low MPV is very characteristic of WAS in boys with thrombocytopenia.

✦ WAS protein expression can be studied by flow cytometry, which is reduced in the majority of patients with WAS.

✦ Genetic testing to look for mutations in the WAS gene is diagnostic.

Immunological phenotype: Immunoglobulin levels are highly variable in patients with WAS. High IgE is noted in the majority of patients. Lymphocyte subsets (T, B and NK cells)—normal.

Treatment: Monthly IVIg and cotrimoxazole prophylaxis. BMT is curative.

Phagocytic Defects

Chronic Granulomatous Disease (CGD)

The inability of neutrophils to kill intracellular organisms.

Etiology: Defect in NADPH oxidase.

Pathogenesis: NADPH oxidase consists of 5 subunits (gp91phox, p47phox, p67phox, p40phox, p22phox). This enzyme is essential for the production of superoxide ions (free radicals) necessary to kill intracellular organisms (bacteria and fungi). Defect in any of the subunits can cause CGD (Table 28.3). Patients with CGD are pre-disposed to infections with catalase-positive organisms.

Clinical presentation
+ CGD is characterized by recurrent suppurative infections—suppurative lymphadenitis, empyema, lung abscess, liver abscess, osteomyelitis, etc.
+ Non-resolving pneumonia is a common presentation. Organisms— catalase positive organisms—*Staphylococcus aureus, Klebsiella, Pseudomonas, Acinetobacter, Serratia, Burkholderia.*
+ Infections with unusual organisms—*Burkholderia, Pseudomonas, Serratia,* and unusual fungi warrant evaluation for CGD.
+ Can present with blood in stools-colitis.

Diagnosis: Diagnosis of CGD can be easily established by an abnormal nitroblue tetrazolium test (NBT) and dihydrorhodamine test (DHR). The principles of these tests have been explained in detail in Chapter 19. Genetic testing can be performed by NGS (next generation sequencing), however, mutations in the NCF1 gene (coding for p47phox) can be missed by NGS as the NCF1 gene has a large pseudogene.

Immunological phenotype: CGD is characterized by hypergamma-globulinemia. Lymphocyte subset (T, B and NK cells) is normal. Abnormal NBT and DHR tests are diagnostic.

Treatment
a. In the presence of fever, empirical treatment covering *S aureus* warranted. Every attempt must be made to isolate organisms. Poly-microbial infections are possible.
b. Cotrimoxazole and itraconazole prophylaxis.
c. HSCT is curative.

Table 28.3: CGD—pattern of inheritance, genes and proteins involved

Inheritance	Gene	Protein
X-linked	CYBB	gp91phox
AR	CYBA	p22phox
AR	NCF1	p47phox
AR	NCF2	p67phox
AR	NCF4	p40phox

X-linked CGD is the most common form in the European and North American studies, however, AR CGD due to p47phox is the most common variety in India (AR diseases are more common in our set-up due to high rates of consanguinity).

Leukocyte Adhesion Deficiency (LAD)

Neutrophils fail to reach the infected tissues.

Etiology: Defect in adhesion of neutrophils to the endothelium, due to a deficiency of adhesion molecule (integrins/selectins).
+ LAD type 1: ITGB2 mutation, CD18 deficiency
+ LAD type 2: Mutation in GDP-fucose transporter gene, CD15 deficiency
+ LAD type 3: Mutation in FERMT3 gene. Defect in the activation of integrin

Pathogenesis: Neutrophils extravasate to the site of infection and handle the pathogens. This process involves attachment of neutrophils to the endothelium, diapedesis, chemotaxis, and phagocytosis. Neutrophils express integrins and selectins which are essential for binding of neutrophils to the endothelium and defect in these molecules is known to cause LAD. As neutrophils fail to extravasate, very high neutrophil counts are noted in this setting.
+ LAD type 2 is a glycosylation defect and is characterized by the Bombay blood group.
+ LAD type 3 has a defect in activation of integrin. Neutrophils cannot adhere to the endothelium. It also results in defective platelet aggregation and children present with Glanzmann thromboasthenia—like bleeding.

Clinical Features
+ *"Very high neutrophil count is a clinical clue."*
+ Delayed fall of the umbilical cord, recurrent pneumonia, ear infections non-healing ulcers, perianal lesions, gingivitis.
+ Type 2 is also characterized by neurological involvement—microcephaly, seizures, short stature, and abnormal facies.

Diagnosis
+ *Type 1:* Absent CD18 expression on neutrophils (flow cytometry). Confirmation by genetic testing.
+ *Type 2:* Bombay blood group; absent CD15 expression on neutrophils (flow cytometry). Confirmation by genetic testing.
+ *Type 3:* Bleeding manifestations and recurrent infections. Diagnosis—genetic testing.

Treatment
+ Severe forms of LAD (CD18 expression <1%)—bone marrow transplant.
+ Milder forms—antibiotic prophylaxis (CD18 expression >1% and <30%)

Complement Defects

C1q Deficiency

Etiology: Deficiency of C1q, autosomal recessive inheritance.

Pathogenesis: C1q is the first complement protein in the classical pathway. This pathway is activated by an antigen–antibody complex. The result is the formation of the membrane attack complex (MAC) which kills the pathogen. C1q is an opsonin and clears encapsulated bacteria and immune complexes. Deficiency in C1q results in infections with encapsulated bacteria and autoimmune disorders.

Clinical features
a. Early-onset lupus (below the age of 5)
b. Infections with encapsulated bacteria (*S pneumonia, H influenza, etc.)*

Diagnosis: In children with early-onset lupus (onset below the age of 5), one must look for an underlying genetic disorder. CH50 is markedly reduced in patients with C1q deficiency. Confirmatory tests—C1q levels and genetic testing.

Treatment: Lupus must be treated on the standard protocol. FFP infusions can be tried as it provides C1q. Bone marrow transplant is curative (C1q is produced by bone marrow stromal cells, unlike other complement proteins, which are produced by the liver).

Note

1. Recurrent neisserial meningitis—terminal complement pathway defect (C5–C9 deficiency)
2. Defects in complement regulatory proteins—atypical hemolytic uremic syndrome (HUS), e.g. factor H deficiency

Did you know?

+ The number of publications on primary immune deficiencies in India has increased by 10 times in the last decade!
+ A refection of rising awareness and better diagnostic facilities!

SUGGESTED READING

1. Candotti F. Clinical Manifestations and Pathophysiological Mechanisms of the Wiskott-Aldrich Syndrome. *J Clin Immunol*. 2018; 38(1):13–27.

2. Jindal AK, Pilania RK, Rawat A, Singh S. Primary Immunodeficiency Disorders in India-A Situational Review. *Front Immunol*. 2017; 8:714.

3. Ming JE, Stiehm ER, Graham JM Jr. Syndromic immunodeficiencies: genetic syndromes associated with immune abnormalities. *Crit Rev Clin Lab Sci*. 2003; 40(6):587–642.

4. Schröder-Braunstein J, Kirschfink M. Complement deficiencies and dysregulation: Pathophysiological consequences, modern analysis, and clinical management. *Mol Immunol*. 2019; 114:299–311.

5. Yazdani R, Fekrvand S, Shahkarami S, et al. The hyper-IgM syndromes: Epidemiology, pathogenesis, clinical manifestations, diagnosis and management. *Clin Immunol*. 2019; 198:19–30.

Patient Advocacy Groups

When patients are diagnosed with uncommon or rare diseases, they often feel isolated and lost. A patient organization that is formed by such families is a great source of relief and comfort in this setting. We are fortunate to have **Primary Immunodeficiency Patients' Welfare Society (PIDPWS)**, a non-profit organization based in Bangalore that has been formed by the families of patients with PID. They have been effortlessly trying to help newly diagnosed families with PID to cope up with the challenges of the condition and support them emotionally and at places, financially. They also conduct educational programs and meetings on PID to raise awareness amongst medical fraternity and the lay public. The government of Karnataka now provides free intravenous immunoglobulin infusions to all children with PID, thanks to the tireless efforts of the PIDPWS. This society shall play a very crucial role in the days to come, in the field of PID. Very much like in the West, such societies can help many needy families by providing social, emotional and financial support. They can fund research and produce an enormous impact on the science of PID.

For more details of the society, please refer to the following website—www.pidindia.net

Office address of the Society:
I.e. No.25A, HHS/HMS Complex,
Cubbonpet Main Road,
Bangalore 560002;
Mob No: +91 9448147224

Did you know?

Several state governments (Punjab, Haryana, Rajasthan, Karnataka, etc.) provide free monthly immunoglobulin injections to children with PIDs.

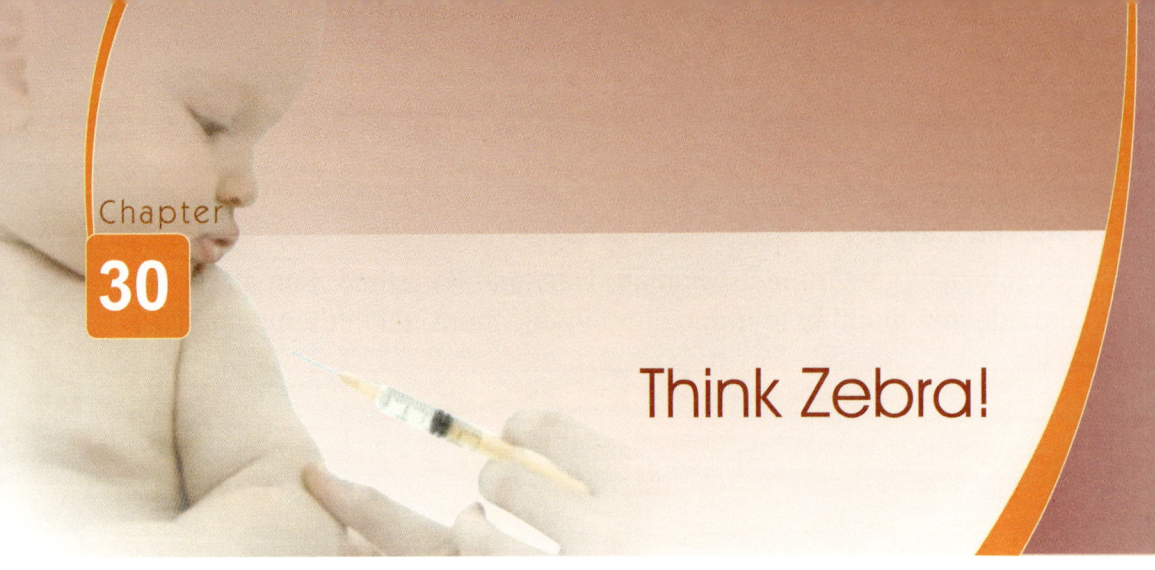

Think Zebra!

If the readers of this book have anytime heard me speaking on PID, in a medical conference or on the YouTube videos, you would have noted the title of my talk—"Primary Immune Deficiency: Think Zebra!" You must be wondering what's Zebra in this conversation?

During our medical training, we are often made to think of common diseases while analysing our patients. This approach may be the correct in many ways and we may diagnose unresolved cases by this approach, but not always! Thinking 'out of the box' is an art and must be learnt. When you hear hoofbeats, you often think of horses. 'Horses'—the common diseases. But it would be wise to think of 'Zebras' as well! 'Zebras'—the PIDs!!!

PIDs are the Zebras of the medical world and unless you think about them, you don't see them, you don't diagnose them! It is high time we think of zebras in our day-to-day medical practice. "THINK ZEBRA" is the logo of the "Immune Deficiency Foundation" (IDF), an organization based in New York, United States (Fig. 30.1)

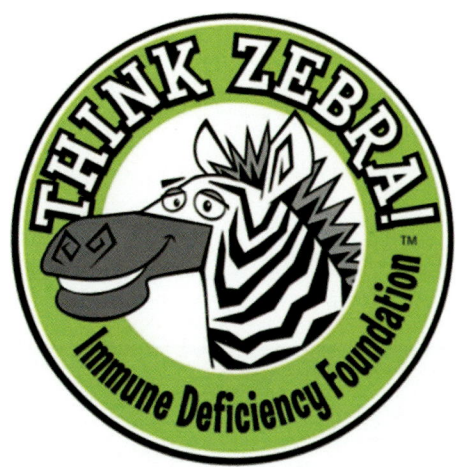

Fig. 30.1: Logo of the Immune Deficiency Foundation

On the scientific front, the field of PID is expanding at an exponential rate with newer diseases being added to the book of PID every now and then. On the clinical front, several patients are now being diagnosed, thanks to the rising awareness and better diagnostic facilities. For a better understanding of this interesting subject, I have prepared brief video-snippets with case-based discussion on various types of PID. These videos are available on YouTube and can be accessed with the following links.

1. Approach to B-cell defects
   https://www.youtube.com/watch?v=_XzHl5Kpmyo

2. Approach to phagocytic defects part 1
   https://www.youtube.com/watch?v=TvJuCXFoJAc

3. Approach to phagocytic defects part 2
   https://www.youtube.com/watch?v=iut3Fj9W3sU&feature=youtube

4. Approach to T-cell defects
   https://www.youtube.com/watch?v=gZeCa_GfSoQ

5. Is my child's immunity low? A video for parents.
   https://www.youtube.com/watch?v=RrE0h4GKVW0

I sincerely hope this booklet and these videos would guide clinicians in diagnosing patients with PID and in the process, many families would receive timely treatment.

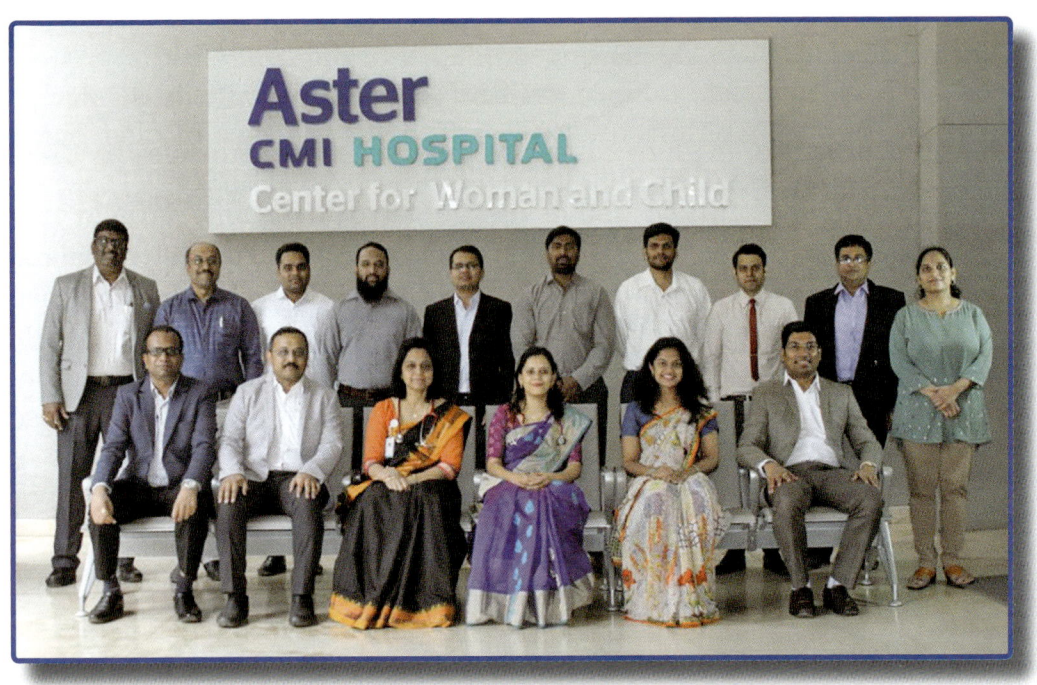

Best wishes from the Department of Pediatrics,
Aster CMI Hospital, Bangalore, India

Index